Dietary approaches to Irritable Bowel Sy

Müge Arslan

# Dietary approaches to Irritable Bowel Syndrome (IBS)

**PETER LANG**

**Bibliographic Information published by the Deutsche Nationalbibliothek**
The Deutsche Nationalbibliothek lists this publication in the Deutsche
Nationalbibliografie; detailed bibliographic data is available online at
http://dnb.d-nb.de.

**Library of Congress Cataloging-in-Publication Data**
A CIP catalog record for this book has been applied for at the Library of Congress.

Cover illustration © iStock.com/Rimma_Bondarenko

ISBN 978-3-631-78674-1 (Print)
E-ISBN 978-3-631-78979-7 (E-PDF)
E-ISBN 978-3-631-78980-3 (EPUB)
E-ISBN 978-3-631-78981-0 (MOBI)
DOI 10.3726/b15606

© Peter Lang GmbH
Internationaler Verlag der Wissenschaften
Berlin 2019
All rights reserved.

Peter Lang – Berlin · Bern · Bruxelles · New York · Oxford · Warszawa · Wien

This publication has been peer reviewed.

www.peterlang.com

*For My family...*

# Preface

Throughout my career track as a nutritionist, I have pushed people to eat more balanced diets and to live healthier and higher quality lives and during this process, I have observed that gastrointestinal issues are among the most common problems my patients suffer from. Intestines (and the gut microbiota), often referred to as the "real brain" of the body, has been implicated in a wide range of diseases, including obesity and diet has a direct impact on intestinal health.

While bloating, gas and constipation seem like routine, everyday symptoms, one can't deny the significant societal burden they impart partly through their effect on the quality of life and partly through the medical and surgical costs they incur by patients desperate to get rid of them.

As I compiled my extensive research on Irritable Bowel Syndrome (IBS) in this book, my goal was to share professional know-how with my colleagues and other healthcare professionals to help them make more informed medical decisions on behalf of their patients. For me, sharing knowledge is an important and meaningful privilege and only those words that have been shared become immortal. I thank everyone who patiently stood by me through this process, who shared their knowledge love and experiences, and those who took the time to carefully read this book.

*Assistant Professor Müge Arslan, Ph.D.*

# Contents

# Introduction

Nutrition is one of the most important factors defining human life, and its impacts start in the womb. It is a process that includes the intake, digestion, absorption and metabolisation of nutrients necessary for the body to function. In short, nutrition is a function impacting all stages of human life, from food production to cellular use. Human health is affected by several factors, such as nutrition, inheritance and environmental conditions, while nutrition is the most significant among all. Hence, from infancy into adolescence and adulthood, healthy eating habits have a very important role in maintaining good health, preventing diseases and ensuring a high quality of life.

Nutrition also has an impact on social well-being. Insufficient or unbalanced nutrition not only leads to health problems, but also increases social burden by reducing work performance and increasing workplace accidents and relevant health costs. Therefore, an adequate, balanced and healthy diet is of great importance for a healthy society. An adequate diet consists of sufficient intake of energy, nutrients and other bioactive substances that are required by human body. A balanced diet is the balanced consumption of balanced meals based on nutrients. Healthy nutrition is the proper selection and use of nutrients, with knowledge on their potential harms during production, storage, preparation and cooking.When examined in this respect, nutrition has functions in the maintenance of many metabolic processes, such as those of the immune, endocrinological, physiological, and gastrointestinal systems. It is possible to have a healthy gastrointestinal system with optimal digestive and excretion processes.

Nutrients have a significant role in the whole digestive process. The presence of nutrients in the gastrointestinal tract affects gastrointestinal motility, sensitivity, the barrier function and intestinal microbiotics. The formation of atypical modulator mechanisms of the intestine as a response to the stimulation of intestinal receptors results in irritable bowel syndromes (IBS). The type of diet that is adopted has a role in the exacerbation of IBS symptoms as well as its treatment.

# 1 Irritable Bowel Syndrome (IBS) and FODMAP Diet

## 1.1 Irritable Bowel Syndrome (IBS)

Irritable bowel syndrome has a long history.

IBS is a chronic, functional gastrointestinal (GI) disorder characterised by recurrent abdominal pain, bloating, and changes in the amount and quality of faeces. It is one of the most commonly seen GI disorders, with a global prevalence of 10 %–20 %. (1,2) IBS has been reported with differences between phenotypes in epidemiology, risk factors and different regions throughout the world.(3) The prevalence of IBS is higher in industrialised countries in Western Europe, USA, Canada, Australia and New Zealand compared to developing countries in Asia, the Middle East, South America and Africa.(4)

The pathogenesis of this disorder is extremely complex and probably multifactorial (abnormalities in motility, internal organ sensitivity, brain-intestine interaction, intestine permeability, immune system activation, neuroendocrine function, gallbladder acids and intestinal microbioma).(5)

Although IBS patients occasionally have food allergies, some studies reported that the exacerbation of GI symptoms is related to certain carbohydrates, fruit and vegetables, dairy products and legumes. (6)

Symptoms include bloating, abdominal pain, constipation and diarrhoea. Internal organ sensitivity, low-grade inflammation and inability to control flatulence are in the etiology of IBS.(7,8)

IBS was first defined in 1989 with the principles in the Rome I guidelines, and through development, the understanding moved to "the absence of structural disease" and "gastrointestinal function disorder," according to the latest Rome IV criteria published in May 2016. In Rome IV, the concept was expanded with impaired motility, visceral hypersensitivity, altered mucosal and immune function, altered intestine microbiota, and the impaired intestine-brain interaction related to the altered central nervous system process.

Based on the Rome criteria, IBS is defined as recurrent abdominal pain related to changes in defecation behaviour.

There are 4 sub-types of IBS: (9)

1. **IBS with predominant constipation** (hard or lumpy stools ≥ 25 % / loose or watery stools, bowel movements < 25 %);
2. **IBS with predominant diarrhoea** (loose or watery stools ≥ 25 % / hard or lumpy stools, bowel movements <5 %);
3. **Mixed IBS** (hard or lumpy stools ≥ 25 % / loose or watery stools, ≥25 % bowel movements);
4. **Unclassified IBS**

Due to lack of specific diagnostic symptoms, IBS is still diagnosed from symptomatic criteria, or the Rome criteria (the latest version, Rome IV). (9) Various methods from manometry, colonoscopy and enteroclysis, to stool cultures and blood tests are helpful in diagnosing this disease. Routine laboratory studies, such as full blood count and blood enzyme panels, are considered routine applications for IBS.

Diagnostic evaluation depends on whether the predominant symptom is constipation or diarrhoea. Psychological factors and nutritional habits are used as screening tools for IBS. (10,11)

Although the basis of IBS is complex, there is increasing evidence to show that factors such as food, gallbladder acids, antibiotics and infections, gender and psychosocial events are all contributors.(12) These factors, which have been previously genetically or epigenetically determined, may lead to microbiota changes caused by abnormal sensorimotor outcomes, neuroendocrine reactions and changes in the intestinal epithelial barrier via local and brain immune activation, associated with the duration and severity of symptoms(13,14,15) (Fig. 1)

IBS is related to a change in intestinal microbiota characterised by increased rates of proteobacteria and actinobacteria and decreased rates of firmicutes and intestinal microbiota. While there is usually an increase in certain bacteria strains (i.e. escherichia, fusobacterium) causing pro-inflammatory effects in IBS patients, there is a significant decrease in anti-inflammatory strains (i.e. faecalibacterium, roseburia). (16) IBS patients have a different microbial composition than patients in recovery. Previous studies have shown lower levels of Clostridium coccoides, Clostridium leptum, Faecalibacterium prausnitzii and Bifidobacterium in IBS patients.(17)

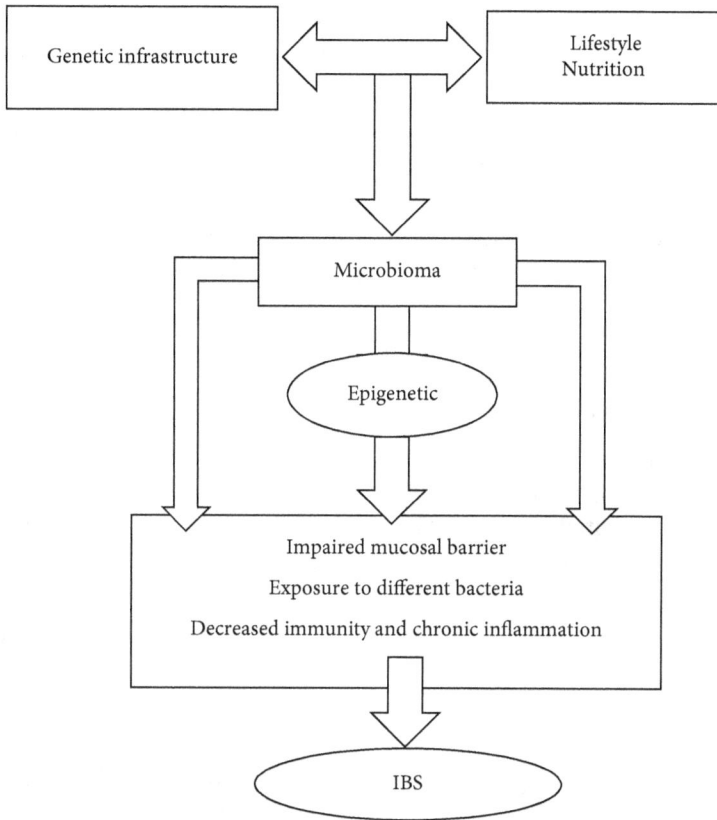

Fig. 1: The pathological and physiological mechanisms suggested for inflammatory bowel disease (IBD). There is a complexity of the assumed role of epigenetics on the interaction between the microbiota with genetic and lifestyle factors and the immune system as well as the mucosal barrier. (171)

There are few studies that investigate changes in microbioma during the course of the disease. In a study in the Netherlands that monitored 10 Chrohn's disease patients and 9 ulcerative colitis patients, no general changes in microbial composition or variations were reported. In another study in Spain, where 18 ulcerative colitis patients were monitored for a year, a uniform increase in Faecalibacterium prausnitzii was observed in patients in recovery, whereas levels remained low in those whose conditions worsened again. Intestinal colonisation starts immediately after birth, and rather than genetic predisposition, it is impacted in the early stages of life by the type of birth, infant diet (i.e. mother's milk vs formula) and hygiene. While use of drugs, stress and toxins (e.g. tobacco) play an important role in the modulation of microbioma composition, several other factors can potentially affect the composition of microbiota. (18,19,20)

Recent research has shed light on the role of epigenetic modifications (i.e. non-coding RNAs and DNA methylation) in defining the molecular basis of IBS. (21,22) These studies have shown that genetics alone may not explain the onset of IBS. A meta-analysis of GWAS studies estimated that sensitivity to ulcerative colitis explained only 16 % of its contribution to ulcerative colitis. In this context, it is suggested that gene-environment interaction plays an important role in the pathogenesis of IBS, and that epigenetics could present new information. Therefore, epigenetic factors have been presented to mediate interactions between the environment and genome; thusly, new information has been provided in the pathogenesis of IBS. (21,23,24) In previous studies, a differentiated expression of specific microRNAs in colonic mucosa samples of IBS patients compared to the mucosa of control patients was reported.

MicroRNAs identified in peripheral blood have also been recommended as new biomarkers in the development of the disease. (25) The latest data has shown that microRNAs are involved in the differential regulation of cytokines and in the immune response to the spread of bacteria. In Th17 cells, in particular, microRNA disregulation plays a role in IBS. MicroRNAs have been shown in ulcerative colitis (UC) and in the regulation of the integrity of the intestinal barrier.(25,26) DNA methylation inscriptions have been described more recently for UC and Chrohn's disease. However, the systematic correlation of changes in DNA methylation and gene expression has not been clearly shown. (27)

In addition, a series of studies point out the role of diet in IBS, which can be explained with atypical modulator mechanisms of the intestine as a response to the stimulation of intestine receptors modulated by nutrients. The presence of nutrients in the GI tract has an effect on GI motility, sensitivity, barrier function and intestinal microbiota. (28) Similarly, food hypersensitivity and food intolerance underlie IBS pathogenesis, but there is lack of high-quality evidence to support these mechanisms. (29)

Hypersensitivity to some food products causes low-grade intestinal inflammation, increased permeability of the epithelial barrier and visceral hypersensitivity. Bioactive chemicals in food (e.g. salicylates) may trigger and contribute to GI symptoms in IBS causing visceral hypersensitivity following possible chronic exposure. (28,30)

Luminal distension, nutrition and short-chain carbohydrates have been proposed as another mechanism causing symptoms in IBS, which may increase luminal water retention and gas production, and could thereby lead to bloating, pain and increased visceral hypersensitivity. (27,30) Furthermore, GI symptoms have been related to specific foods in at least 2 of every 3 IBS patients, and this demonstrates the importance of diet management in IBS treatment. (30,31) This has been supported by the focus on concerns related to food and GI problems, typical dietary recommendations in IBS and specific foods to be avoided, but usually patients have been left with an unnecessarily restricted diet which has resulted in inadequate nutrition. It is therefore of the greatest importance that dieticians and doctors present nutrition recommendations in detail to IBS patients. (32,33)

## 1.2  The First Line of Dietary Approach in IBS

Diet and lifestyle recommendations are crucial for managing IBS. In addition to typical recommendations around restricting intake of potential diet triggers, such as alcohol, caffeine, spicy food and fat, regular nutritional habits must be monitored. Patient must stay hydrated and should exercise regularly. (34,35)

### 1.2.1  Nutritional Habits

Several studies suggest that IBS patients have irregular eating habits compared to healthy individuals, which can affect colonic motility and therefore contribute to IBS symptoms. (36,37) Similarly, according to another study that compares obese and non-obese females, the risk of IBS is twice to four times greater in obese females, and that higher food consumption can contribute to GI symptoms.(38)

Food choices and amounts have a significant effect on IBS. Therefore, both patients and healthcare professionals must be well-informed on nutritional habits, food choices and amounts in order to reduce the symptoms of IBS.

According to scientific literature on IBS, recommendations for nutritional habits, food choices and amounts are as follows: IBS patients should have regular meals (breakfast, lunch and dinner, with appropriate food choices for these meals), food should be well-chewed and not swallowed quickly and meals should be eaten while seated. (34,35,39)

## 1.2.2 Spicy Food Consumption

Several IBS patients reported that eating spicy food triggers GI symptoms, such as abdominal pain and gastroesophageal reflux. (31,40,41)

In a recent, large, cross-sectional study of adults in Iran, where mean daily pepper consumption (i.e. 2.5–8 g per person) is much greater than that in Europe and USA (i.e. 0.05–0.5 gr per person), it was reported that the tendency for IBS increased significantly in females consuming spicy food at least ten times a week.(42)

Known as the active component in red pepper, capsaicin causes these effects on the GI tract. (43,44) In healthy individuals, capsaicin accelerates GI passage mediated by vanilloid type-1 (TRPV1), which has temporary receptor potential, causing pain and burning. In impairments characterised by visceral hypersensitivity, including those reported in IBS patients, an increase in the number of TRPV1 receptors has been observed.(45,46) Some studies show that abdominal pain and burning exacerbate with addition of capsaicin. (47,80) However, it must be noted that spices were used at high doses in these studies and there was no data regarding habitual consumption of spicy food or its role in the treatment. There are also studies showing that chronic consumption of red pepper has a beneficial effect on IBS. Some studies also suggest that the analgesic effect of red pepper works as a pain killer during the first couple of weeks of treatment, while the impact is temporary. (81)

**Recommendations for consumption of spicy food for IBS patients, according to scientific literature:**

✓ The intake of spicy food must be assessed in IBS patients, and if related to IBS symptoms, consumption should be restricted. (34)
✓ Other spicy food (e.g. fructants in onions and garlic) should also be assessed. (34)

### 1.2.3  Fat Intake

A significant proportion of IBS patients show symptoms in response to high fat food. (41,50,51) One of the strictest dietary approaches taken to correct the symptoms of IBS patients is to completely avoid fats. (52) Laboratory-based studies have shown that duodenal lipids impair intestinal gas clearance, causing gas retention and bloating, thereby inhibiting movement in the small intestine. (53,54) Duodenal lipids increase in colorectal hypersensitivity with the perception of increasing rectal distension in IBS patients. (55,56) Despite these laboratory studies, there is little evidence associating dietary fat intake with IBS.

There are no randomised, controlled trials supporting that a reduction in fat intake in particular leads to an improvement in IBS symptoms. (33,57) In a previous cohort study, no difference was determined in fat intake between IBS patients and a control group. Recent research has also shown a hypothetically positive effect of dietary fat in IBS. (58,59) There are studies showing that polyunsaturated fatty acids and metabolites could show beneficial effects on intestinal inflammation. However, to be able to state a definite effect, there is need for further research of polyunsaturated fatty acid supplementation in IBS patients. (59)

**Recommendations for fat intake for IBS patients, according to scientific literature:**

✓ If IBS symptoms are seen during fat intake or before or after a meal, intake must be provided according to principles of healthy nutrition, and fat intake must be evaluated. According to the FAO / WHO dietary recommendations, total fat intake of an adult should be between 15 % and 30 %–35 % of total energy. (60)

✓ It is recommended that the fat intake of IBS patients is limited to 40–50 g per day.(39)

### 1.2.4  Intake of Milk and Dairy Products

Milk and dairy products contain lactose, which is a disaccharide not well-digested by majority of humans. (61) This explains the low level of lactase enzyme in the human intestinal mucosa. (39)When milk is consumed, undigested lactose is broken down into short-chain fatty acids by intestinal flora and causes the GI symptom of gas (e.g. hydrogen).(62) The typical GI complaints of lactose intolerance are similar to those of IBS, including abdominal discomfort, bloating and diarrhoea. (61) Many IBS patients have similar symptoms related to milk and dairy product consumption, although not all of these have been confirmed by means of standard tests. (63,64)

Some studies have reported that IBS symptoms in a significant proportion of patients have improved in response to a lactose-free diet. Despite these findings, not all these experiments have been blinded or controlled. The improvement of symptoms may be related to lactase deficiency in some patients. (39) In a small, double-blind, placebo-controlled study, lactase support was reported to ameliorate IBS symptoms. It is also possible to hypothesise that milk components other than lactose could play a role in IBS. For example, it was suggested in one study that milk intolerance in some cases could be related to the ingestion of protein A1-casein. During digestion, this protein is known to express β-casomorphine 7, which shows GI effects. (65) There is a need for further studies to clarify the role of milk and dairy products in IBS.

**Recommendations for milk and dairy products intake for IBS patients according to scientific literature:**

✓ A low lactose diet should be recommended to IBS patients only if a positive lactose hydrogen breath test is present. (34)
✓ If IBS patients want to follow a dairy-free diet, they should be informed that there is no viable evidence that this diet improves the symptoms. Patients should also be informed that a diet low in calcium could lead to insufficient daily calcium intake. (34)
✓ For IBS patients with suspected milk sensitivity, and for whom the lactose hydrogen breath test is not possible or not appropriate, a low-lactose diet can be recommended for a trial period. (34)

### 1.2.5 Predominantly Plant Nutritional Intake

Vegetarianism is a plant-based diet that includes different diet types depending on consumption of animal byproducts, such as eggs and milk. (82) Previous studies draw connections between vegetarianism and several health benefits, such as reduced risk of ischaemic heart disease mortality, general incidence of cancer and development of type-2 DM. (83,84) A semi-vegetarian diet (SVD) was evaluated over two years in CD patients, and there was a more significant decrease in symptoms for those on SVD compared to those eating both meat and vegetables.(85) SVD is a lacto-ovo vegetarian diet with restricted intake of animal-origin protein, which emphasizes the daily intake of fruit and vegetables, brown rice and grains. Fish consumption is permitted once a week, meat once every two weeks and unlimited eggs and dairy products. More than half the patients on SVD who participated in the study showed a decrease in symptoms and normal concentration of C-reactive protein (CRP) during the final check-in. The researchers estimated that long-term continuation of SVD and normalisation of CRP levels would lower the risk of the disease worsening. The Mediterranean diet, which is widely accepted as a valid dietary intervention, can be beneficial in managing various pathologies and reducing general mortality. (86,87) The Mediterranean diet comprises of plant-origin nutrients (e.g. grains, vegetables, fruits, pulses, nuts, seeds, olives), a moderate amount of olive oil, high amounts of fish and seafood, eggs, poultry and dairy products (cheese, yogurt), small amounts of red meat, and a moderate amount of alcohol (especially wine with meals).(88) In a study of CD patients, those who followed the Mediterranean diet for six weeks showed a decrease in inflammatory biomarkers (e.g. CRP) and a tendency for the intestinal microbiology to return to normal. (89)

## 1.2.6 Animal Protein Intake

In a non-randomised interventional study, the effect of animal protein taken with the diet in general was examined on the maintenance of reduction of IBS symptoms. In 183 ulcerative colitis (UC) patients consuming high levels of meat and meat products (processed meat), an increased risk of the possibility of the disease worsening was predicted. (48) There is a need for additional studies to be able to fully clarify its effect. (49)

## 1.2.7 Dietary Fibre Intake

In some IBS patients, fibre consumption can exacerbate symptoms and increase abdominal pain and bloating. (69,70) The effect of fibre in IBS has been much debated in respect to soluble and insoluble fibre, with recommendations to increase intake of soluble fibre and decrease insoluble fibre consumption. However, this approach may no longer be appropriate as both properties are in fibrous foods, such as psyllium and oat flakes and most plant-origin foods contain a mixture of soluble and insoluble fibre. (34,71)

A more suitable approach is based on classification of fibre, not just based on solubility but also on fermentation, viscosity and gel formation: insoluble, slightly fermented (wheat bran), soluble, unseen, easily fermented (inulin), soluble viscous/gel-forming, easily fermented (β-glucan) and soluble, viscous/gel-forming unfermented (psyllium). While easily fermented fibres lead to rapid gas formation, slightly fermented or unfermented fibres generally do not cause gas formation. (72) As there have been few studies on this subject, the role of fibre in IBS is still a matter of debate.

In a systematic review of 12 randomised, controlled studies, 621 subjects were evaluated with the symptom score or a global evaluation and neither soluble or insoluble fibre was found to have any beneficial effect on the improvement of abdominal pain.(73) In contrast, a more recent systematic review and meta-analysis of 14 randomised controlled trials including 96 patients reported that soluble fibre, such as psyllium, could have some beneficial effects on IBS; and, that insoluble fibre, such as bran, was of no benefit and could even exacerbate symptoms. These data, supported by information related to the fermentability of fibres, showed that soluble viscous dark fibres with a low fermentation rate (e.g. psyllium) could be the most appropriate both for constipation and for diarrhoea in IBS patients.(71)

The addition of cotton seed to the diet can be useful in the management of constipation. Cotton seed is a rich source of dietary fibre and, according to previous studies, ground cotton seed has been reported to improve constipation and abdominal pain, as well as gradually reduce bloating in IBS-C over a period of 3 months. (34)

**Recommendations for dietary fibre intake for IBS patients based on scientific literature:**

✓ There is no definitive evidence about the optimal amount of fibre in IBS, but according to previous studies, total dietary fibre (natural intake and supplementation) of 20–30 g per day is considered appropriate. (74)

However, it is not recommended for IBS patients to increase intake of wheat bran above normal nutritional habits. (34)

✓ IBS-C patients should be advised to follow a 3-month trial diet where they should consume two tablespoons (150 ml/tablespoon) of cotton seed supplement mixed with a liquid. Improvements in GI symptoms obtained with cotton seed supplementation can last for up to 6 months. (34)

## 1.2.8 Caffeine Intake

Previous studies have shown that coffee, especially caffeinated coffee, increases gastric acid secretion and colonic motor activity in healthy individuals. (71,75) It has also been reported that coffee stimulates rectosigmoid motor activity and has a laxative effect in sensitive individuals. (34) However, the role of caffeine in IBS is not very clear. (39) Several studies have shown a relationship between the symptoms of IBS patients and coffee and tea, although it has also been reported that drinking coffee is not as widespread in IBS patients as it is in healthy individuals. (32,50,76) Furthermore, it is not clear whether a lower amount of caffeine intake would provide better clinical results. (66,77)

**Recommendations for caffeine intake for IBS patients based on scientific literature:**

✓ Caffeine intake should be evaluated in IBS patients and, if associated with symptoms, majority of adults should be restricted to 400 mg caffeine per day. (34)

In addition to coffee and tea, other sources of caffeine, such as energy drinks, soft drinks, dark chocolate and some non-prescription analgesics, as well as their amounts should also be examined. (71)

## 1.2.9 Alcohol Consumption

Alcohol is known to affect GI system motility, absorption and permeability. (77) However, there is limited evidence related to alcohol consumption in IBS. (39) According to studies evaluating self-declared food intolerance, alcohol has a role in GI symptoms. (7,32) In contrast, population-based studies do not show any correlation between alcohol consumption and IBS.(66,68) However, in females with IBS, GI symptoms, such as abdominal pain and diarrhoea, have been tied to consumption of more than four servings of alcohol per day as opposed to low (e.g. 1 serving per day) or moderate consumption (e.g. 2-3 servings per day). (77) There is a clear need for further randomised trials to clarify the relationship between alcohol consumption and IBS.

**Recommendations for alcohol consumption for IBS patients, according to scientific literature:**

✓ Alcohol consumption should be decreased and alcohol intake should be evaluated if GI symptoms improve, (34)
✓ The safe alcohol consumption limit recommended to IBS patients is less than two days per week. (34,78)
✓ In general, the safe alcohol limit is defined as a maximum of one serving per day for females and two servings for males. (79)
✓ A unit of alcohol is defined as 12oz for beer (5 % alcohol) 5oz for wine (12 % alcohol); and, 1.5 oz for 80° distilled alcohol (40 % alcohol). (79)

### 1.2.10 Fluid Intake

Although there is no evidence in scientific studies related to the effect of fluid intake in IBS, current dietary recommendations promote fluid intake of 1.5–3 L per day. To increase the frequency of defecation and reduce the need for laxatives in IBS-C, sufficient fluid intake is recommended. Water and other caffeine-free drinks, such as herbal teas, are suggested for IBS patients. Carbonated water and other carbonated drinks should be avoided by IBS patients as they may cause symptoms. (82,83)

**Recommendations for fluid consumption for IBS patients based on scientific literature:**

✓ IBS patients should be advised to drink 1.5–3L of fluid per day (approximately 35ml/kg), especially water or caffeine-free, non-alcoholic and non-carbonated drinks (e.g. herbal teas). (80,81)

### 1.2.11 Physical Activity

If diet is supported with physical activity in management of IBS, healthier and more successful result can be achieved. This is due to physical activity serving a basic complementary function to diet. Regular exercising is good for health, and recent data has emphasised the positive effects on IBS patients. Some studies have reported that light physical activity has reduced IBS symptoms, cleaned the intestines, and reduced bloating and constipation. Yoga has also been shown to improve IBS symptoms in both adolescents and adults. (89,90)

The mechanisms underlying the benefits of physical activity in IBS are a reduction in splanchnic blood flow, neuroimmuno-endocrine transformations, an increase in GI motility and reduction in mechanical jumps during movement. The effect of exercise on psychological symptoms is accepted as a potential mechanism, and studies have reported positive effects on quality of life, fatigue, anxiety and depression in IBS patients following a moderate increase in physical activity. However, it must also be taken into consideration that physical activity, (88) especially intense exercise, could make IBS symptoms worse. While moderate physical exercise (e.g. fast-paced walking) has been reported to improve intestinal clearance time, intense physical activity (e.g. running), however, could have a stress effect on the intestine and could result in severe diarrhoea. (92,93)

**Recommendations for physical activity for IBS patients based on scientific literature:**

✓ Physical activity levels of IBS patients should be evaluated ideally using the General Practice Physical Activity Questionnaire. IBS patients who do not exercise regularly should be advised to exercise more regularly. (35)

✓ Moderate level physical activity, such as yoga, walking, cycling or swimming for at least 30 minutes per day for 5 days a week is recommended for IBS patients. Approximately two-thirds of IBS patients perceive GI symptoms to be related to food. Carbohydrates that have not been fully absorbed (lactose in dairy products, beans, onion, cabbage, apples and wheat), fatty food, coffee, alcohol and spicy food reportedly trigger and exacerbate GI symptoms. (35,78)

Several previous studies have focused on elimination or strict exclusion diets to research the role of food intolerance in IBS patients. These studies have all provided different results according to the type of food excluded, the duration of exclusion and the type of participant. (41,94)

Lactose malabsorption due to lactase deficiency is known to cause abdominal pain, bloating and loose bowel movements .(95) Some studies have investigated the role of a low-lactose diet in IBS management. In a study of 22 IBS patients, lactose malabsorption was determined in 27 % with a positive lactose hydrogen breath test, but following a low-lactose diet, the symptoms were observed to have been alleviated in only 9 (39 %) patients.(96) In contrast, another study involving IBS patients with lactose malabsorption reported a significant decrease in symptoms with a lactose-restricted diet, but no improvement was seen in IBS patients who did not have lactose malabsorption. Therefore, although there are conflicting results about lactose malabsorption and restriction, a lactose-restricted diet should be attempted for patients with lactose malabsorption but other diet restrictions may also be necessary. (97)

### 1.2.12 Probiotics

Supplementation is another diet treatment that has been intensively studied both in IBS and several other conditions. However, as each probiotic could have different properties including varying effects on cytokines, host microbiota and other potential targets, the effects are possibly specific to each probiotic rather than in a whole classification. (98) A range of dietary applications have been studied in IBS treatment including high-fibre diets, gluten-free diets, reduced-lactose diets and low-fat diets.

Another recent dietary approach is FODMAP, which has researched the relationship between IBS and fermentable, oligosaccharide, disaccharide, monosaccharide and polyols foodstuffs. (99)

## 1.3 Second Stage Approach of Low-FODMAP Diet

The term FODMAP was first used by researchers at Monash University in Australia to define a collection of poorly absorbed, short-chain, fermentable carbohydrates which are natural components of many foodstuffs: (100)

- Fructans (including inulins) and oligosaccharides containing galacto-oligosaccharides,
- Lactose and sucrose containing disaccharides,
- Fructose containing monosaccharides,
- Sorbitol and mannitol containing polyols.

FODMAPs (fermentable, oligosaccharide, disaccharide, monosaccharide, and polyols) are a group of short-chain carbohydrates which are poorly absorbed in the GI tract.

Monosaccharide, fructose, oligosaccharide and fructant are a part of FODMAPs. Lactose, which is a disaccharide, is found in milk and dairy products. Polyols are sugar alcohols found in certain fruits, such as peaches and plums. Sugar alcohols such as sorbitol, lactitol and xylitol, which are widely found in products not containing sugar. (101,102)

---

**FODMAP** concept

- Fermentable
- Oligosaccharide          - FOS, GOS, fructants, rafinose, inulin
- Disaccharide             - lactose (galactose-glucose)
                           - sucrose (glucose-fructose)
- Monosaccharide           - fructose

AND
- Polyols                  - sorbitol, mannitol, xylitol, maltitol

---

Key characteristics are poor absorption in the small intestine and rapid fermentation in the colon.

At least 70 % of polyols cannot be absorbed in healthy individuals. (101) These highly osmotic materials are rapidly fermented by bacteria. FODMAPs may be the cause of GI symptoms through immune-mediated pathways, lumen distension or by direct movement of the FODMAPs themselves. Many IBS patients have visceral hypersensitivity which may be triggered by sudden lumen distension. Some individuals may be even more sensitive than others to some FODMAP groups.(104,105) Böhn et al. examined the self-reported diet intolerance of IBS patients, reporting a high food sensitivity to FODMAPs in 70 % of patients, sensitivity to dairy products in 49 % (high in lactose), sensitivity to beans (galactane) in 36 %, and sensitivity to plums (fructose+polyols) in 23 %. (94)

Previous studies have shown that consensus has been reached on the subject of the necessity of the second stage of IBS diet management to include dietary applications such as low FODMAP, which have been developed to relieve symptoms when IBS symptoms persist even when general diet and lifestyle recommendations are followed some of the foods have high and low amounts of fodmap content (106)

Tab. 1: High and Low FODMAP Foods (172)

| Sugar type | High FODMAP foods | Low FODMAP foods |
| --- | --- | --- |
| Oligosaccharides | **FOS**<br><br>Grains: wheat, rye and barley-based products<br><br>Vegetables: onion, garlic, artichoke, leek, beetroot, cabbage<br><br>Fruit: watermelon, peach, date, prune, nectarine, and mostly dry fruits<br><br>**GOS**<br>Legumes: lima beans, dried beans, soy beans<br><br>Vegetables: beetroot, peas | Fruit: banana, strawberry, (not blackberries), grapes, lemon, mandarin, orange, kiwi, pineapple, passionfruit, rhubarb<br><br>Vegetables: red pepper, bok choi, green beans, beetroot, cucumber, carrot, celery roots, eggplants, lettuce, Jerusalem artichoke, tomatoes, zucchini<br><br>Grains: non-wheat grains/flour, gluten-free bread or grain products and quinoa<br><br>Dairy products: lactose-free milk, almond or rice-based milk, yogurt and ice-cream, hard cheese, Feta cheese and cottage cheese<br><br>Fruit: banana, grapes, melon, kiwi, lemon, linden berries, mandarin, orange, passionfruit, strawberries (not blackberries) |
| Disaccharides | **Lactose**<br>Dairy products: cow and goat milk and yogurt | Sweeteners: maple syrup and golden syrup |
| Monosaccharides | **Fructose (glucose)**<br>Fruits: Apple, pear, watermelon, mango, cherries, thyme honey and fruits high in fructose<br><br>Sweeteners: high fructose corn syrup<br><br>Vegetables: asparagus, peas | Sweeteners: maple syrup and sugar (sucrose)<br><br>Fruit: banana, grapes, melon, kiwi, lemon, mandarin, orange, passionfruit |

Tab. 1:    Continued

| Sugar type | High FODMAP foods | Low FODMAP foods |
|---|---|---|
| Polyols | **Sorbitol**<br>Fruits: apple, pear, avocado, apricot, blackberries, nectarine, peach, plum, prune, watermelon<br><br>**Mannitol**<br>Vegetables: sweet potato, mushrooms, cauliflower, peas | |

Notes: Data obtained from Monash University. Low FODMAP Diet Application. (http://www.med.monash.edu/cecs/gastro/fodmap/. Android version, 26 August 2015.72)

Abbreviations: FODMAP = **fermentable, oligosaccharide, disaccharide, monosaccharide and polyols**, FOS =fructo-oligosaccharides; GOS, galacto-oligosaccharides.

## Alternative High and Low FODMAP Sources
## HIGH FODMAPs
### Fructants:

✓ Whole grains, such as bread, pasta, couscous,
✓ Onions, shallots, spring onions, garlic,
✓ Barley,
✓ Brussels sprouts, cabbage, broccoli,
✓ Pistachio, artichoke, inulin, chicory root

### Galactanes:

✓ Soy milk, soy protein isolate,
✓ Miso (Japanese),
✓ Vegetable burger,
✓ Dry beans, peas, lentils,
✓ Butter,
✓ Lima beans, hummus,
✓ Coffee exceeding 1 cup per day

### Lactose:

✓ Soft cheese, including Ricotta, cream cheese
✓ Milk, cream, yogurt, butter, ice cream

**Polyols:**

✓ Artificial sweeteners (xylotol, sorbitol etc)
✓ Apple, plum, cherries, pear
✓ Cauliflower, sweetcorn, peas, mushrooms

## LOW FODMAPs

**Fruits:**

✓ Orange, sugar-free cornelian cherry, strawberries, melon, lemon, linden berries, plum

**Vegetables:**

✓ Peas, celery roots, carrots, tomatoes, spinach, lettuce, green pepper, green beans, beansprouts, turnip, cucumber

**Dairy Products**

✓ Hard cheese, including Kasseri (or Kasar), Swiss cheese and Parmesan.
✓ Lactose, and sugar-free yogurt, lactose-free milk

**Meat, Dry Fruits and Nuts**

✓ All plain processed meats, peanut butter (sweetened with high fructose corn syrup)
✓ Eggs,
✓ Almonds and walnuts in small amounts, tofu

**Grains**

✓ Rice (all types),
✓ Gluten and rye-free bread,
✓ Oat flakes, corn, oat rice, brown wheat or quinoa grains, corn tortilla, semolina, popcorn, potatoes, quinoa

## 1.3.1 The FODMAP Mechanism

The FODMAP mechanism in triggering symptoms is very likely due to the stimulation of mechanical receptors as a response to luminal bloating from the osmotic effect, especially in the small intestine, from a combination of the increased amount of luminal water content, mostly from carbon dioxide and hydrogen gas expression, and the amount of poorly absorbed fructose, polyols and lactose.(107,108) This type of stimulation can lead to increased signalling, which can be interpreted as pain or bloating, while the effect on movement with potential changes in the intestinal structure is a response in the diaphragm and anterior abdominal wall, causing increased abdominal bloating. Although FODMAPs in large amounts (e.g., lactulose) can cause diarrhoea, the amount required is generally much more than that consumed in the diet.

This is important because some researchers believe that a low-FODMAP diet is best for those with diarrhoea-predominant IBS (IBS-D). However, this belief is not consistent with data obtained from controlled, clinical studies, which have shown that while these applications do not make improvements in constipation-predominant IBS (IBS-C) patients, bowel clearance and the water content of faeces change at a very small amount in response to diet. (109) Bowel movements can be affected by the short-chain fatty acids (SCFA) expressed from the fermentation of FODMAP's. There has been no direct evaluation of whether or not visceral sensitivity is affected by changes in FODMAP consumption. SCFAs may change this, and visceral sensitivity may be altered with the expression of histamine as a neuroinflammatory response including mast cell activation. As a change in FODMAP intake alters the intestinal microbioma, other pathogenic mechanisms may play a role in symptom modulation.

There are weak reports showing that some patients have been more sensitive to FODMAP exposure following a period of restriction, suggesting that because of the temporary effect of bloating caused by increased fibre content, adaptation of the microbiota or enteric nervous system could be significant. Therefore, although the reduction of luminal distension continues to be an important mechanism inducing FODMAP symptoms, close proximals have started to be resolved and other mechanisms could also play an important role. (110,111)

## 1.3.2 The Application of a Low FODMAP Diet

The direct and indirect effects of FODMAPs on the intestinal microbiota, intestinal barrier, intestinal response and visceral sensitivity are known to include symptom formation.(112) Studies have shown that there could be a positive effect of a low FODMAP diet on IBS symptoms. (109,113,114) It is thought that the main effect mechanism of low FODMAP diets is a reduction in small intestine absorption of osmotically active SCFAs and this reduces intestinal water content, causing effects reducing colonic fermentation and gas production. (115,116)

Recent studies have shown that low-FODMAP diets decrease the levels of pro-inflammatory interleukines, IL-6 and IL-8, faecal bacteria (Actinobacteria, Bifidobacterium and Faecalibacterium prausnitzii), total faecal SCFAs and n-butyric acid levels. (117,118) Although the response to a low FODMAP diet may be related to patient demographics, microbioma components, metabolism and factors associated with the IBS subtype, there have been no large-scale studies providing definitive results. (119,120)

Given the high prevalence of IBS, observed deficiencies in the training of dieticians in the use of low FODMAP diets and the limited availability of reliable FODMAP data present a significant obstacle to its use in clinical applications. (121) Furthermore, both printed and online material on this diet is lacking.

There have been no studies of material printed about the diet or of what can be learned from information on the internet. (122) The Monash University Low-FODMAP Diet smartphone app has facilitated access to current FODMAP composition. This app includes detailed and ongoing food analyses of foodstuffs in 10 countries and 4 continents. (123)

### 1.3.3 Low FODMAP Diet Compared to Alternative Therapies

Evidence obtained from randomised studies has consistently shown that a low FODMAP diet is superior to placebo approaches (only diet or observation). While it is important to define its efficacy compared to other IBS therapies, to date no randomised, placebo-controlled studies have been performed to measure the efficacy of any other diet therapy. Instead, the low FODMAP diet has generally been compared directly and indirectly to other diet strategies and non-pharmacological approaches directed at IBS patients. (124) Three studies compared the low FODMAP approach with the local version of the diet as described in the UK National Institute for Health and Care Excellence (NICE) guidelines.

The first of these studies was a non-randomised comparison of a low-FODMAP approach applied for a predetermined period within the UK. (125) The study can be evaluated as an examination of two competitive approaches. The 76 % response rate of patients on a low FODMAP diet outperformed the NICE diet which had a 54 % response rate. The second study, which was a recently conducted randomised study in Sweden, reported similar responses to the low FODMAP diet as to a traditional IBS diet. (113) The traditional diet included recommendations regarding eating habits (regular meals, not eating too much at once, and eating slowly), the selection of food (reduced fat intake, spicy food, coffee, alcohol, onions, beans, and cabbage), and the avoidance of carbonated drinks, gum and artificial sweeteners ending in "-ol".

The traditional diet included reduced intake of FODMAPs, but according to an evaluation performed on a measured database, the measured intakes surprisingly only showed a small drop in FODMAPs. A low FODMAP diet was basically effective from lactose intake rather than the intake of other FODMAPs (the Swedish study showed that there could be minimal effect). Both interventions were administered by dieticians and were equally effective.

Therefore, 19 (57 %) of the 33 patients who completed the low FODMAP diet and 17 (50 %) of 34 patients who completed the traditional IBS diet, with a minimum 50 % reduction in 4 weeks at the IBS Symptom Severity Score have generated a response.

However, the 57 % response to the low-FODMAP diet was far below what was expected, as previous observational and randomised studies had reported rates of 68 %–86 %. (107,126) In the third study, conducted in the USA, the patient population was restricted to diarrhoea-predominant IBS (IBS-D) patients and the traditional diet was changed from NICE guidelines with no restriction of high FODMAP content foods. (127) Although the primary outcome (general satisfaction) of traditional IBS diet and low FODMAP diets were not different, many secondary outcome analyses, especially abdominal pain and swelling, showed significant benefits of the low FODMAP diet. The traditional IBS diet only partially reduced FODMAP intake. Limited evidence has shown that with the gradual re-addition of FODMAPs the continuous restriction of only a mild FODMAP, at least 75 % of patients could maintain good symptom control. This raises the question of whether or not a strict elimination stage is necessary. (128)

In a randomised, controlled study of 87 IBS patients following high and low FODMAP diets, rye bread was the only nutritional difference, with symptoms then evaluated. Although the inclusion of the bread to the low FODMAP diet reduced some symptoms and respiratory hydrogen production, the patients did not generally show a full recovery. That study provided evidence for a more extensive change in the diet rather than only limiting the diet to foods containing high FODMAPs. (129)

### 1.3.4 Hypnotherapy for the Intestines

Many randomised, controlled studies have been conducted on the effects of hypnotherapy on IBS patients.(130) In a recent randomised clinical trial, the short and long-term effects of bowel-directed hypnotherapy were compared with the low FODMAP diet and showed similar sustained effects in relieving gastrointestinal symptoms.(128) A total of 74 patients were randomly separated into groups receiving hypnotherapy, diet, or both treatments. In the 6th week, 72 % of patients in the hypnotherapy group, 71 % of patients in the diet group and 73 % of patients that received both therapies reported clinically significant improvements in gastrointestinal symptoms. This observed improvement continued 6 months after the initiation of treatment in 74 %, 82 % and 54 % of patients respectively. This shows that hypnotherapy targeting the intestines could have an effect at similar rates as those observed for the low FODMAP diet. Although a significant improvement in quality of life was reported in all the groups of IBS patients, a higher level of improvement in the psychological indexes were obtained through hypnotherapy. It was concluded that when a specialist is available to provide hypnotherapy for the intestines, this modality can be considered as an alternative to diet. (124)

### 1.3.5 Gluten-free Diet

Wheat is accepted as one of the most common foodstuffs causing abdominal pain, bloating and/or changes in bowel habits. (131) In a study conducted in Australia involving 1184 adults, it was found that 8 % of the participants avoided wheat or followed a gluten-free diet to relieve symptoms.(132)

One of the most debated points concerning which wheat components are responsible for the clinical effect of protein (gluten) and carbohydrate (basic FODMAPs), as indigestible oligosaccharides, fructants and galacto-oligosaccharides are found together in wheat, rye and barley. (131,133)

Although no comparative study was performed between the low FODMAP diet and GFD, the observational report of the benefits of GFD in diarrhoeal IBS (IBS-D) patients had a similar response to low FODMAP diets. (134) The majority of patients continued with a GFD and during an 18-month follow-up period, they reported that they were still following the diet and that their symptoms had improved.

Similarly, 13 obese patients with IBS-D following a very low carbohydrate diet (reduction of FODMAPs and gluten containing only 20 g of carbohydrate per day for 4 weeks) reported a decrease in stool frequency and texture, and improvement in pain scores and quality of life. (135) Although these observations were impressive, they are not helpful in explaining whether symptoms improve, are not associated with a placebo, or are due to the absence of gluten or a reduction in FODMAP intake with the avoidance of foods containing grain. In only one randomised controlled trial, the gluten-containing diet in IBS patients was compared with a gluten-free diet.(136) In a 4-week evaluation of 45 patients with IBS-D, a reduction in the frequency of less than 1 defecation per day in a gluten-containing diet was observed and or no change in transition. (133)

Patients with IBS-like symptoms, which may or may not be extra-intestinal symptoms, apart from celiac disease and wheat allergy, are said to have non-celiac gluten sensitivity (NCGS). (137) Some of them may have undiagnosed celiac disease. Uncontrolled symptoms are seen in approximately 25 % of patients despite the avoidance of gluten, and another food intolerance has been determined in 65 % of patients.(138) In a cross-sectional, controlled, randomised study, gastrointestinal symptoms improved in all 36 patients who were started on a low FODMAP diet at early stages, with no recurrence or exacerbation of symptoms, especially in patients on a low-gluten FODMAP diet.(139)

These data indicate that low FODMAP associated with wheat, rye and barley avoidance has resulted in partial responses to symptoms in high FODMAP, suggesting that this response can be further improved by FODMAP restriction. In another randomised, controlled study, by rarely determining gluten to be responsible in the diet, a similar gluten-specific deficiency was observed at the onset of symptoms in self-reports of the vast majority of NCGS patients. (140,141) In most IBS patients, it is important to differentiate between gluten or FODMAP intolerance.

To help define trigger foods and the amounts causing symptoms, clinicians can decrease diet restrictions to a minimum, can provide appropriate substitutions for excluded foods and can optimise the range of the diet. Thus, risk factors such as micronutrient deficiencies, low-fibre diet, dysbiosis and irregular nutrition, which are associated with a low-FODMAP diet and GFD, can be minimised. (138,142)

### 1.3.6 Predictors of Response to Symptoms

Biomarkers and clinical characteristics that predict the individual response of a patient showing sensitivity to a low-FODMAP diet and certain FODMAP types (e.g. glucose, lactose, sorbitol, mannitol, and excessive fructose in oligosaccharides) allow clinicians to select the most appropriate and least interventional treatment options. To date, there have been no data showing that the problems related to FODMAPs in general or specific FODMAPs directly influence the symptom forms. (124)

### 1.3.7 Hydrogen Breath Test

Despite uncertainties in the methodology, poor repeatability of results and difficulties in interpretation, the hydrogen breath test continues to be widely used in clinical applications to direct diet management. (107) The need to restrict each FODMAP is based on whether or not they are connected to symptoms and whether or not specific FODMAPs are absorbed after the consumption of sugar (i.e., an increase in hydrogen in the breath). However, as oligosaccharides are always malabsorbed, the hydrogen breath test may not be of potential benefit. This tool is applied more to lactose to determine the presence of hypolactase, and to slowly absorbed FODMAPs (fructose, sorbitol, mannitol), to determine whether any of the swallowed doses have entered the colon.

The degree of malabsorption depends on the digested FODMAP dose (e.g. while 50 gr fructose can be malabsorbed in 80 % of patients, malabsorption may only be 10 % in a 25 gr dose), the time of passage through the small intestine, and a congenital reduced absorption capacity.(143) The determination of fructose malabsorption has low repeatability, which shows that results obtained at any point within a time period may not reflect the underlying absorption capacity.(144) An increase seen in the hydrogen breath test does not show any correlation between impaired absorption of fructose, mannitol and sorbitol, and GI symptoms.(144,145) This may possibly be due to the osmotic effect of the slow absorption of FODMAPs in the lumen of the small intestine. Diet adjustments are only one aspect of IBS management strategy. IBS management is multi-model and diet is only a strategy. Previous studies have reported that a low-FODMAP diet can be applied without prior hydrogen breath testing, and specific sensitivities can be determined at the stage of reforming the diet. (124)

### 1.3.8 Stool Microbioma Analysis

Recently, there has been great interest in the microbiome and metabolite profile examination. A study of a paediatric population evaluated whether or not there was a symptomatic response to a low-FODMAP diet, based on pain frequency and microbiota that were estimated at the beginning of the study. (120) This was a randomised, double-blind, cross-sectional study of children given a high or low FODMAP content diet for 2 days. To determine predictors before feeding, patients were separated into groups based on the frequency of pain as those who responded, did not respond, or responded to a placebo during the application of the 2 diets. Those who responded were found to have an increase in abundant taxons such as Bacteroides, Ruminococcus and Faecalibacterium prausnitzii, which are known to have a greater carbohydrate fermentation capacity. This finding was observed to be compatible with the hypothesis maintaining the effect of a low-FODMAP diet is related to a decrease in intestinal lumen distension and patients with sacrocrolytic potential enriched microbiota can obtain the utmost benefit from a reduction in the substrates which can be fermented in the diet. No such relationship has been found in adults to date. There is a need for more data from parallel arm experiments. (118)

## 1.4 Low FODMAP Diet in Children with Functional Gastrointestinal Disorders

According to the Rome III criteria, approximately 5 % of school-age children have IBS.(146,147) Reports of childhood IBS show low quality of life, increased risk of depression and increased social isolation and school absence in affected children. (148,149) The cost of diagnosis has been estimated to be 6,000 USD per child. (150) An increase in the disease burden makes it likely that paediatric cases will continue into adulthood. (151)

Although there is a popular belief that symptom development is related to food intolerance, and even though children have reported that symptoms are exacerbated by certain foods, there are very few paediatric controlled studies. However, recent evidence has emerged showing that low-FODMAP diets have been taken into consideration when treating children with IBS. (126) Chumpitazi *et al.* conducted a double-blind, randomised, controlled study of 52 children, aged 7–17, with IBS.(120) After basic data was gathered over 7 days, children were provided with a low-FODMAP diet or a moderate FODMAP diet for 2 days. The children then completed a 5-day detoxification period; a daily reduction of abdominal pain was observed in both groups. In adults, the maximum response to a reduction in FODMAP intake is 7 days. Therefore, an intervention over a longer time frame could allow for the emergence of a greater effect. (109)

### 1.4.1 Malabsorbed Carbohydrates and Functional Abdominal Pain

Despite all the studies involving children and the effects of a low-FODMAP diet, some poorly absorbed carbohydrates, such as lactose, fructose and sorbitol, have a long-term role in the pathogenesis and treatment of paediatric functional gastrointestinal disease (FGID). In 1985, Hyams and Leichtner reported that children with non-specific diarrhoea completely recovered after the exclusion of apple juice from the diet; thus concluding that excessive amounts of apple juice caused non-specific diarrhoea in young children. (152) This finding emphasised that modern feeding practices could have an important role in the pathogenesis and treatment of FGID.

Furthermore, it must be considered whether or not the basic nutritional recommendations for a varied and balanced diet (i.e., consumption at sufficient and non-excessive amounts of each of the 5 food groups) are sufficient to regain normal gastrointestinal functions. Hyams and Leichtner also reported an increase in respirated hydrogen in children following the consumption of apple juice. This observation of carbohydrate malabsorption has become a focus of research related to functional GI symptoms in adults and children. The contribution of fructose, lactose and/or sorbitol to functional abdominal pain has been shown in open, non-controlled studies of children.

In a study of 32 children with functional abdominal pain, there was a positive hydrogen breath test for fructose malabsorption in 28 %, while in 81 % of these patients, symptoms rapidly recovered with a fructose-restricted diet and a significant decrease was reported in abdominal pain and bloating 2 months after the first breath test.(153) In another study of a cohort of 222 children with abdominal pain, 55 % had a positive breath test for fructose malabsorption, while 77 % showed clinical improvement after 2 months on a low fructose diet.(154) Wintermeyer *et al.* reported that 42 % of 117 children had a positive hydrogen breath test for fructose malabsorption, of which 75 followed a low-fructose diet for 4 weeks under the supervision of a dietician. (155) Pain frequency and severity was observed to have significantly improved in the 2nd week after starting the diet. In another long-term retrospective study involving 118 children with fructose malabsorption, a reduced lactose, fructose and /or sorbitol diet led to a reduction in the vast majority of symptoms and high family satisfaction. (156) However, in these 4 studies, it remains unclear whether the improvement in pain can be directly attributed to fructose or to fructose malabsorption. First, in the absence of a control group, the benefits could be completely related to a placebo effect. Second, the nature of the diet is unspecified; for example, it is not stated whether more than glucose alone was eliminated, whether or not fructose was restricted, or whether or not fructo-oligosaccharides were eliminated. Third, as no dietary change was made for those without fructose malabsorption, the relationship of the efficacy with the presence of fructose malabsorption could not be evaluated. Finally, the restriction of polyols (found in fruit and fruit juices) could have contributed to this positive effect. Nevertheless, the studies support the theory that changing the intake of poorly absorbed short-chain carbohydrates could be of therapeutic benefit.(124)

## 1.4.2 Hydrogen Breath Test in Children

Studies performed on children assume a positive hydrogen breath test as a predictor of response to an elimination diet. However, the diagnostic value of the fructose hydrogen breath test in children is a matter of debate. First, the capacity to absorb fructose increases up to the age of 10, which is important for the results and interpretation of the test performance in young children. (157) Second, as stated above, adult studies have shown that hydrogen breath tests cannot be reproduced. (144) In a blind, randomised, controlled study of 103 children with functional abdominal pain and the application of a positive breath test, a low-fructose diet was not predicted to give a response to abdominal pain. (158) Finally, lactose, a fructose and/or sorbitol malabsorption diagnosis with a positive hydrogen breath test can lead to the child being labelled with a specific food intolerance. Lactose, fructose and/or sorbitol malabsorption is seen at a similar frequency in healthy individuals as in IBS patients. (159) Visceral hypersensitivity in IBS makes this malabsorption related to symptom management, while acceptance of unnecessary diagnostic tests can be reduced and a functional diagnosis, such as IBS, can be made. (160) It is important to evaluate whether small children with IBS are consuming a high FODMAP diet with excessive amounts of fruit/fruit products, milk/dairy products and wheat/wheat products. In addition, to reduce FODMAP dietary intake to reach the resolution of symptoms, it is important to evaluate whether wheat, dairy products and fruit portions could be normalised with limitations. (124)

A low-FODMAP diet is not a life-time diet. This dietary approach is related to the application of a suitable diet for the individual, and a re-introduction of nutritional components following the monitoring of tolerance to foods rich in FODMAP and a follow-up of symptoms.(161)

**Steps to be followed in the FODMAP Diet:**

**1. Low FODMAP diet**
For 2-6 weeks, the removal of high FODMAP foods from the diet and nutrition is applied with low-FODMAP foods. (161)

↓

**2. The addition of FODMAP foods to the diet**
At 8-12 weeks, the introduction of FODMAP foods, one by one, over 3 days. Through an observation of tolerance, the amount of FODMAP nutrition is increased every day. (161)

↓

**Tab. 2:** Points of Importance in the Diet Manipulation of Children with Gastrointestinal Symptoms (173)

---

A functional GI disorder diagnosis must be made and, to determine specific food intolerances in children, symptoms should be managed rather than reliance on the hydrogen breath test.

---

Recommendations to be initially given to children with IBS;

- Encouraging regular, sufficient and balanced nutritional intake including consumption of each of the 5 food groups. Further encouraging regular water intake.
- Encouraging regular bowel movements as children can confuse abdominal pain with the feeling of dangerous bowel movement. A dialogue should be established with the school to ensure that the child is prepared to use the toilet, not only during breaks, but also during class.

Attention to a low-FODMAP diet in children with persistent IBS symptoms is of value, but only;

- Under the supervision of a dietary specialist
- When there is low risk of eating disorders
- When feeding difficulties, such as food refusal or food selectivity, are at the lowest level so that foods in the low-FODMAP diet will be accepted.

When a low-FODMAP diet is successful, an ideal program should be applied after ≤6 weeks to reduce restrictions to a minimum according to tolerance. The aim of this program is;

- To develop the ability of the child to cope psychosocially
- To prevent the child from distancing him/herself from food
- To minimalise the effect of the reduced dietary prebiotics on the intestinal microbiota

If unsuccessful, FODMAP restriction should not be continued.

Each child exposed to FODMAP restrictions must be re-evaluated at regular intervals (e.g., every 3 or 6 months)

- To monitor nutritional adequacy and growth
- To monitor for nutritional deficiencies
- Regular re-structuring of FODMAP restrictions must be ensured and high FODMAP foods can be re-introduced, according to tolerance. When there is a reduced capacity for fructose absorption in young children, the tolerance levels can change (i.e., increase) as the child grows.

---

FODMAP; fermentable, oligosaccharide, disaccharide, monosaccharide and polyol IBS; irritable bowel syndrome.

## 3. A personalised FODMAP diet

Patients eventually become aware of which foods they can or cannot tolerate and they then can feed themselves with foods that they find tolerable in the long run. (161)

## 1.5  The Risks of a Low-FODMAP Diet

Although diet therapies are accepted as generally good, there is a risk of side-effects in all therapies; the low-FODMAP diet is no exception. Problems of nutritional deficiencies are always a concern in restrictive diets. For IBS patients following a low-FODMAP diet, 3 problems have been defined. (124)

### 1.5.1  Incorrect Use of the Low-FODMAP Diet

One of the observations, for example, as summarised by the Rome Association, has been that healthcare professionals are using the low-FODMAP diet as a diagnostic test rather than as an approach for a positive diagnosis (personal observations). This is similar to the use of a gluten-free diet by the population in general to diagnose gluten sensitivity. These types of applications are weak approaches because in any patient with intestinal symptoms, these symptoms can potentially improve with reduced FODMAP intake, without any understanding of whether the underlying disease is functional or congenital. As with all therapeutic tools, a low-FODMAP diet must be applied under the right circumstances. (165,166)

### 1.5.2  Changes in Gastrointestinal Microbiota

Fructants and galacto-oligosaccharides have prebiotic actions. Restrictions in the adjustment of a low-FODMAP diet can lead to a reduction in beneficial bacteria. Several studies have shown a relationship between a decrease in the relative abundance of Bifidobacteria in the stool at 3 and 4 weeks of a diet very low in FODMAPs. In a study comparing IBS patients with a healthy control group, a decrease in Bifidobacteria in the IBS patients was observed and a negative correlation was determined between the amount of faecal Bifidobacteria and IBS pain scores.

If there is causality of dysbiosis in IBS (although there is no direct evidence supporting this), there may be a contrary effect of a strict low-FODMAP diet. In addition, there is a significant reduction in absolute and relative numbers of strong butyrate-producing bacteria, and with the strict reduction of FODMAP intake, mucous-destructive bacteria can increase. However, the clinical importance of these changes is unknown. The microbioma of IBS patients have not been examined following the re-inclusion of high-FODMAP foods at levels that are tolerated, since it is recommended that a strict low-FODMAP diet only be followed for 2–6 weeks. Compared to a healthy control group, when it is considered that the microbiota of IBS patients undergo more extensive temporary changes, a greater change is observed in response to dietary alterations. Thus, there is a need for further broader-based studies to demonstrate the real short term and long term effects of a low-FODMAP on the microbiome of patients with IBS.(168)

### 1.5.3 Irregular Meals

Literature points to evidence that patients with GI disorders who have made dietary changes could be at high risk of irregular eating behaviours. Satherley *et al.* reviewed evidence for irregular dietary practices in celiac and IBS patients, and found the prevalence to be similar to that of other healthy control groups in the dietary-controlled group, thus food intake should be monitored continuously. These individuals may feel anxious when preparing food and when confronted with different foodstuff. (169) These types of behaviours have recently been associated with orthorexia nervosa, which is a condition limited by the quality of the diet. This condition is associated with symptoms such as an "obsessive focus on food selection, planning, purchasing, preparation, and consumption. (170) " Food is seen primarily as a source of health rather than one of pleasure, and that an exaggerated belief is accepted that including or excluding food types prevents disease and affects recovery and daily health.(169) These characteristics can be seen in patients who are strongly attached to diet management. The limited evidence in this area states that this condition affects both the physical and psychological welfare of the patient. Regular screening of food pathology, in addition to appropriate referrals, may assist clinicians in recommending alternative therapeutic strategies to patients showing evidence of irregular eating habits. Hypnotherapy, which focuses on diet and restrictive eating practices, can be another option for IBS patients. (124)

## 1.6  An Example of 5-day FODMAP Diet List

### DAY 1

**Breakfast**

- 1 boiled egg
- Tomatoes, cucumbers
- 1 walnut
- 1 thin slice of gluten-free bread

**Snack**

- 2 small mandarin oranges

**Lunch**

- Grilled salmon / boiled broccoli
- Green salad

**Snack**

- 1 carton of lactose-free yogurt

**Dinner**

- 1 plate of green beans
- 1 plate of gluten-free pasta

### DAY 2

**Breakfast**

- 1 thin slice of Cheddar cheese
- 3 olives
- Tomatoes, cucumbers
- 1 thin slice of gluten-free bread

**Snack**

- Almonds (max.15)

**Lunch**

- Grilled chicken with soy sauce
- Green salad

**Snack**

- 1 kiwi fruit

**Dinner**

- Minced meat and aubergine
- 1 cup of lactose-free yogurt
- 1 thin slice of gluten-free bread

## DAY 3

**Breakfast**

- ½ cup of oat flakes + water or lactose-free milk + ½ banana

**Snack**

- 1 handful of hazelnuts (max. 40 gr.)

**Lunch**

- Grilled meat
- Quinoa salad with parmesan cheese

**Snack**

- Orange

**Dinner**

- Gluten-free spaghetti bolognese

## DAY 4

**Breakfast**

- 1 thin slice of goat's cheese
- Tomatoes, cucumber, red-yellow pepper
- Almonds
- 1 thin slice of gluten-free bread

**Snack**

- 1 glass (200ml) of soya milk or lactose-free milk

**Lunch**

- Chicken with mushrooms
- Green salad

**Snack**

- 1 cup of popcorn

**Dinner**

- A zucchini dish
- 1 cup of lactose-free yogurt
- 1 thin slice of gluten-free bread

## DAY 5

**Breakfast**

- Oatflakes with soy milk and berries

**Snack**

- 1 medium-sized orange

**Lunch**

- Grilled turkey
- Arugula salad

**Snack**

- Pumpkin seeds

**Dinner**

- 1 plate of green beans
- 1 cup of lactose-free yogurt
- 1 thin slice of gluten-free bread

# 2 Constipation

## 2.1 The Relationship between IBS and Constipation

IBS is characterised by abdominal pain related to defecation and changes in the frequency and texture of stool, and most IBS patients generally complain of constipation. The Rome III criteria define a sub-type of IBS as predominantly with constipation (IBS-C). IBS and functional constipation (FC) are two functional bowel diseases (FBD). Therefore, in both conditions there is the common thread that the cause cannot be explained by morphological, metabolic or neurological changes that may show up in routine diagnostic techniques. (174)

Although IBS-C and FC are different FBDs from a theoretical aspect, in practice they are very similar and there may even be conditions in which they cannot be differentiated. The primary symptom in both is constipation alongside abdominal bloating/distension. The presence of abdominal pain more than once a week and a temporary relationship of pain with defecation theoretically differentiates IBS-C from FC. Some researchers have considered that, as FC symptoms are similar to those of IBS-C, this reason is false and a patient meeting IBS criteria can be classified as FC.

Previous studies showed that IBS-C has been differentiated from FC by the presence of abdominal pain. In several other studies, the validity of treating IBS-C and FC as different disorders has been questioned. (175,176) These researchers have considered that IBS-C and FC could be part of a continuum that shows differentiation according to the severity of symptoms, while others have differentiated FC subtypes based on the presence or absence of abdominal pain. (177,178)

The Rome III criteria for IBS and FC imply that differences should be found between IBS-C and FC symptoms. (174) An IBS diagnosis requires abdominal pain or discomfort, whereas an FC diagnosis is based on the presence of at least 2 of 6 symptoms (hard stool, infrequent bowel movements, straining, a feeling of not having fully evacuated, a feeling of faecal obstruction, and the need to ease stool output through manipulation). One of these differences in the diagnostic criteria is that the presence of abdominal pain will differentiate the IBS-C from FC and patients with

FC are expected to report more than 6 of the constipation symptoms compared to IBS-C patients.

Wong *et al.* conducted a prolonged follow-up study of 1615 patients in a primary level healthcare institution in the USA, comparing 231 patients with FC according to the Rome III criteria and with 201 patients with IBS-C according to the Rome III criteria.(175) In 89.5 % of the IBS-C group, criteria for FC were met. Following the Rome criteria, it was reported that the two disorders were to be excluded from each other and that the patients were to be followed for one year. At the end of the 1-year follow-up period, it was reported that 40.5 % of the FC group and 25.5 % of the IBS-C group did not have constipation, but in one-third (32 %) of the remaining FC patients, IBS-C or mixed IBS-C criteria were met. Heidelbaugh *et al.* conducted a large-scale, cross-sectional study based on a questionnaire given to 10,030 participants. The results showed that 228 participants met the Rome III criteria for IBS-C and 552 met the criteria for FC. (176) As expected, according to the Rome III diagnostic criteria, the IBS-C group reported more pain and abdominal discomfort than the FC group, but patients in the FC group reported pain on mean 1.2 days per week and abdominal discomfort on mean 1.4 days per week. To further elucidate the overlapping occurrence of symptoms, FC patients were separated into sub-groups of 363 patients with chronic idiopathic constipation with abdominal symptoms (CIC -A; abdominal pain, abdominal discomfort, stomach cramps and/or bloating at least once a week in the previous 12 months) and 189 patients with chronic idiopathic constipation with no abdominal symptoms. The rate of subjects experiencing abdominal discomfort and bloating very frequently or at an extremely uncomfortable level was found to be significantly greater in the CIC-A group than in the IBS-C group, but the result supported that there were no qualitative differences between IBS-C and FC, and all other symptoms (including abdominal pain) were similar. (179) In another study of 125 patients, 49 met both diagnostic criteria. Thus, it was observed that 17 % of all the participants met FC criteria for IBS-C, and 39.2 % met IBS-C criteria for FC. Another clinical-based study in the UK showed that there were significantly conflicting results when the Rome III requirements were ignored in IBS patients not diagnosed with FC. (180)

Several observational studies have supported the hypothesis that IBS-C patients experience more abdominal pain, bloating and discomfort than

FC patients. However, the majority of FC patients have also reported abdominal pain and discomfort. These differences seem to be quantitative rather than qualitative. Moreover, it was observed that patients with FC had more constipation symptoms than IBS-C patients, which suggests that IBS-C and FC cannot be reliably differentiated on the basis of symptoms only. (175,176,178,180) Studies comparing the 2 disorders on quality of life, burden of disease and psychological symptoms scales support the possibility of different points on the same symptom spectrum of IBS-C and FC.

When Wong *et al.* evaluated patients with constipation with a quality of life questionnaire, the quality of life of IBS-C patients was seen to be more impaired than that of FC patients. Drossman *et al.* reported similar results in a study using the Disease Effect Profile. (175,178) In contrast, Zhao *et al.* found no significant difference between IBS-C and FC patients with respect to documented quality of life and symptom severity. (181) Various studies have reported that IBS-C patients have significantly greater anxiety and depression compared to FC patients. (180,181,182,183) It is possible that IBS-C patients seek healthcare services more than FC patients. (176,178,182,183) In addition, FC patients with abdominal pain missed more work days than patients with painless FC, indicating the effect of functional constipation on community burden. (176)

Functional constipation is characterised by straining upon defecation or straining during frequent defecation, or the feeling of not having fully evacuated along with a low frequency of bowel movements. In most cases, no underlying physical cause can be found and this can be accepted as an FBD. (174,184)

The American Gastroenterology Association has classified constipation in 3 groups according to the duration of colonic transit and anorectal function. (185)

## 2.1.1 Normal Transit Constipation

Stool pass normally from the colon: the duration of transit is affected by diet, taking from 20–72 hours depending on drugs used, physical activity level and emotional status.(186) Normal transit constipation is the most widespread form of constipation. This term is sometimes used in place of IBS-C. However, in addition to the main symptom of abdominal pain recovering with defecation, there is occasionally a significant presence of abundant stool. If these symptoms in particular are not definitively identified, it can be difficult to differentiate the 2 conditions.

## 2.1.2 Slow Transit Constipation

The full physiopathology of slow-transit constipation is not known, but a series of underlying causes include changes in colonic muscle or nerve activity, and the loss of enteric neurotransmitters and Cajal interstitial cells. The Cajal interstitial cells are electrically active cells functioning as a pacemaker for the intestines. (187,188) Studies have shown that excessive methane production by colonic bacteria could be responsible for slow transit in some patients.(189)

Opioid-origin constipation is one of the most frequently seen side-effects of opioid analgesic use in patients with chronic opioid use because of cancer, pain other than cancer, and various other reasons. This is a common reason for slow transit and is thought to originate from increased non-propulsive segmental motility and decreased propulsive peristalsis because of μ-opioid receptor activation. The μ-opioid receptors are identified in the myenteric and submucosal plexus of the enteric nerve system in the gastrointestinal system. (190,191)

Slow transit constipation, also known as delayed transit constipation, colonoparesis, colonic inactivity or false obstruction, is defined as a long duration of stool passing through the colon, i.e., more than 5 days. (192) Colonic smooth muscle dysfunction, extended colonic nerve pathways, or both of these, can result in slow colon peristalsis. The use of opioids and factors affecting colonic motility, such as hypothyroidism must be carefully considered in these patients. By reducing intestinal tonus and contractility and thereby prolonging colonic transit, opioids are known to cause constipation. They may also constrict anal sphincters and cause a decrease in rectal function. (193)

## 2.1.3 Evacuation Dysfunction

The pathophysiology has not been fully clarified. Pelvic floor dysfunction or output dysfunction, also known as defensive disorder, is related to defective rectal evacuation. This may result in poor rectal straining strength (slow colonic transit, rectal hyposensitivity), functional resistance to rectal evacuation (high anal resting pressure, anismus, not full relaxation of the anal sphincter, dyssynergic defecation) or structural evacuation obstruction (excessive perineal fall, rectal intussusception). In approximately 50 % of patients with output dysfunction, slow transit constipation is also present. Dyssynergic defecation is the most common output dysfunction disorder and comprises almost half of the cases referred to tertiary level healthcare institutions. A relaxation of <20 % in resting anal sphincter pressure is defined with a paradoxical increase in anal sphincter tone or weak abdominal and pelvic pushing strength.(194)

These definitions have been formed with combined medical views and expert opinions, and patients' opinions related to constipation are also important. (195)

## 2.1.4 The Diagnostic Criteria for Functional Constipation (196)

---

1. 2 or more of the following must be included:
   - Excessive straining in more than 25 % of defecation
   - Lumpy or hard stool in more than 25 % of defecation
   - The feeling of not having fully evacuated in more than 25 % of defecation
   - The feeling of anorectal obstruction/blockage in more than 25 % of defecation
   - Manual manoeuvres in more than 25 % of defecation (e.g., finger in the rectum or applying pelvic pressure)
   - Spontaneous bowel movements <3 times per week
2. Abundant stool seen occasionally without the use of laxatives
3. Insufficient criteria for IBS

---

* The criteria that symptoms should have started at least 6 months before diagnosis and have continued through the previous 3 months

Functional constipation can be categorized into 2 groups, as slow-transit constipation and evacuation disorder. Slow-transit constipation refers to delayed transit of the faecal content in the colon, and is seen more frequently in females. (197)

Other conditions that may cause constipation: (196)

---

- Congenital malformations
- Structural causes or mechanical obstruction
  - ✓ Colon cancer
  - ✓ Benign stricture
  - ✓ Rectocele, enterocele, rectal prolapse
  - ✓ Megacolon
  - ✓ Fissures

- Metabolic
  - ✓ Hypothyroidism, hypercalcemia
  - ✓ Hypokalemia
  - ✓ Uremia
  - ✓ Celiac disease
- Myopathies
  - ✓ Scleroderma
  - ✓ Amyloidosis
- Neuropathies
  - ✓ Spinal injury
  - ✓ Myelomeningocele
  - ✓ Multiple sclerosis
  - ✓ Diabetic neuropathy
  - ✓ Parkinson's disease
- Complications originating from surgery or radiotherapy
- Depression
- Immobility
- Cognitive disorder

## 2.1.5 Pathophysiological Mechanisms

Pathophysiological mechanisms (physiological tests) can differentiate between IBS-C and FC better than symptoms alone. Various pathophysiological mechanisms have been defined for FC including several different paraphysiological mechanisms, paradoxical contraction or insufficient relaxation of pelvic floor muscles during excretion (dyssynergic defecation) and insufficient rectal propulsive force during defecation (known as insufficient rectal propulsion) and, due to reduced high amplitude contractions in the colon, delayed transit through the whole intestine. (198) The balloon evacuation test evaluates the capacity to evacuate a balloon filled with 50 mL water from the rectum within 1–2 mins, and although no specific physiological process is directly measured, it can be helpful in the identification of patients with evacuation disorder. (199) Gastroenterologists see these tests as biomarkers for FC patient groups; based on these assumed pathophysiological mechanisms, patients with chronic constipation are classified as slow-transit constipation or irregular defecation.(200) Despite permanent constipation symptoms, the majority of patients with symptoms compatible with FC do not have delayed transit through the whole intestine or pelvic floor dysfunction. These patients are defined as having normal-transit constipation. (201,202) Unlike those for FC, there is very little consensus on the subject of mechanisms responsible for the symptoms of IBS-C.

Of the widely debated mechanisms, excessive sensitivity to visceral pain is associated with peripheral or central nervous system mechanisms. These include immune mechanisms related to abnormalities in the phasic motility of the small or large intestine, an increased number of mast cells, increased levels of pro-inflammatory cytokines, altered levels of microbiota in the intestines and/or increased mucosal permeability, effects of stress hormones on the intestine, and irregularity in the modulation of perception of visceral pain in the two-way signalling between the intestine and pain. The visceral pain/discomfort threshold has been shown to be the physiological measurement that can most define IBS-C patients, and approximately two-thirds of patients with a clinical diagnosis of IBS-C have an abnormally low pain threshold. (203)

Very few published studies have investigated the basic mechanical differences between IBS-C and FC using a parallel group design of study. The most recent study conducted to compare these groups was by Suttor et al., in which failure to evacuate a water-filled balloon was compared to determine dyssynergy prevalence in 25 FC patients and 25 IBS patients without diarrhoea predominance. However, apart from symptoms, there is no standard for classification of patients as FC or IBS-C; and determining criteria may not be adequate to define overlapping groups. In conclusion, it can be said that when classifying patient groups as IBS-C or FC with comparisons of symptom criteria, the overlap of some physiological symptoms should be expected.

However, the investigators searched for evidence of dyssynergia in patients with at least four symptoms believed to be associated with irregular defecation, particularly in patients with non-diarrhoea-predominant IBS. The possibility of paradoxical contraction has been found to be significantly low in these IBS patients without diarrhoea predominance, and the failure to evacuate the water-filled balloon in the above-mentioned study was found to be significantly greater in the IBS group than in the FC group. The study showed that there was widespread excretion dysfunction in the sub-group of IBS patients, who did not have predominant diarrhoea with evacuation dysfunction symptoms in at least 25 % of bowel movements, but it is not clear what proportion of these patients were of all IBS patients without predominant diarrhoea.

Ansari et al, in India, studied 50 patients with FC and 50 patients with IBS-C and found out that transition times could be faster due to dietary differences and the investigators compared the full bowel passing off time with Sitzmark technique. (204) A tendency for slower transit time was seen in the FC patients (52.2 ± 35.5 hours) compared to the IBS-C patients (41.2 ± 31.6 hours), but the difference was not statistically significant. The rectosigmoid transit time in FC patients was determined to be significantly lower than that of IBS-C patients. In another study, 23 IBS-C patients were compared with 11 FC patients and a healthy control group of 23 subjects. (180) Rectal pain thresholds were found to be significantly lower in the IBS-C group than in the FC group. Although no significant difference was determined in the median colonic transit time, it was found to be longer in both patient groups compared to the healthy control group.

### 2.1.6 Evaluation of Constipation

It is very important for physicians to use treatment tools effectively for constipation. Evaluation of chronic constipation starts with an extensive patient history review and physical examination to exclude secondary constipation. Symptoms, such as unwanted weight loss, blood in the stool, rectal pain and iron deficiency anaemia, should signal alarm; a colonoscopy should be performed for evaluation in respect to malignancy, colitis or other potential colonic abnormalities. (205) A detailed perineal and rectal examination can be helpful in the diagnosis of identified disorders and should include listening during evacuation and evaluation of the anal tone and sphincter. If clinical signs exist, thyroid function tests, electrolyte tests and complete blood count should be given. (206)

Health and social effects of IBS-C and FC are extremely important. In IBS patients, the Health-related Quality of Life (HRQoL) is significantly impaired. (207,208) The costs related to IBS are important role in the economies of countries. In the USA, 3.5 million people visit doctors each year because of this problem, representing a cost of 20 billion USD per year.(209) In Europe, data obtained from Spain in particular have shown an increase in direct and indirect costs for IBS-C patients. For FC patients, it is estimated that there is a deterioration in academic or professional performance and effects on daily life in 69 % of cases, while in severe cases, absence (mean 2.4 days/month) and lower productivity at work have been demonstrated. (210)

Constipation with an estimated worldwide prevalence of 1 % to 8 % is a widespread gastrointestinal disorder, characterised by wide geographical variations and entailing great costs.(211)

## 2.1.7 Treatment

There are pharmacological and non-pharmacological treatment methods for constipation. The drugs used in pharmacological treatment of constipation and associated side-effects are listed below. (212)

| Agent | Typical dose * | Time to onset | Side-effects |
|---|---|---|---|
| **Increasing volume** | | | |
| • Methylcellulose powder | 19 g /day | 12–72 hours | None in comparison with placebo. |
| • Polycarbofil (Fibercon) tablets | 1250 mg, 1-4 times per day | 12–72 hours | None recorded. |
| • Psyllium (Metamucil) powder | 1 teaspoon or 1 packet, 1-3 times per day | 12–24 hours | Bloating, abdominal distension at 4 %–18 % |
| **Osmotic laxatives** | | | |
| • Lactulose solution | 15–30 mL/day | 24–48 hours | Bloating and cramps at the rate of 20 %; nausea |
| • Magnesium citrate solution | 150–300 mL, as a single dose or short-term daily dose | 30 min - 6 hours | Magnesium increase causing paraesthesia hypotension, respiratory depression. |
| • Magnesium hydroxide suspension | 30–60 mL/day | 30 min - 6 hours | Magnesium increase causing paraesthesia hypotension, respiratory depression. |
| • Polyethylene glycol (Miralax) powder | 17 g/day | 24–48 hours | No side-effects recorded. |
| • Sorbitol solution | 2–3 tablespoons, as a single dose or short-term daily dose | 24–48 hours | Bloating, cramps and nausea |
| **Stool softener** | | | |
| • Docusate sodium (Colace) capsules | 100 mg, 2 times per day | 24–48 hours | No side-effects recorded |

| Agent | Typical dose * | Time to onset | Side-effects |
|---|---|---|---|
| **Stimulating laxatives** | | | |
| • Bisacodyl (Dulcolax) tablets | 5–15 mg/day | 6–10 hours | Diarrhoea and abdominal pain in the 1st week at 56 %, and in the 4th week at 5 %. |
| • Senna Tablets | 15 mg/day | 6–12 hours | Abdominal pain 12 % |
| **Chloride channel activators** | | | |
| • Lubiprostone (Amitiza)† capsules | 24 mcg, 2 times per day | Within 24 hours | Nausea 18 % |
| **Peripheral effect mu-opioid antagonists** | | | |
| • Methylnaltrexone (Relistor)‡ solution | Subcutaneous injection according to body weight, 1–2 times per day | 30–60 mins | Diarrhoea 8 % Abdominal pain 13 % |
| **Other** | | | |
| • Linaklotid (Linzess) † capsules | 145 mcg/day | ----- | Diarrhoea 16 % |

Non-pharmacological treatment consists of diet and lifestyle changes, and is traditionally accepted as the first step in a comprehensive treatment program for an effective management of constipation. (213)

**Requirements for a nutritionally balanced diet for the prevention and treatment of constipation:**

✓ **Fibre** intake of 30 g per day is recommended through gradual increases. (214,215) This goal can be achieved with addition of different amounts of bran, and more fruit, vegetables and hazelnuts in the diet. In elderly patients, especially those with heart and kidney diseases, increases in fluid intake must be monitored.(215) In a classic study, it was reported that this approach stabilised colon transit time in geriatric constipation but without any evident improvement in symptoms. (216) In contrast, a recent, small-scale study of 23 elderly females with constipation reported a significant improvement in both parameters with diet and lifestyle changes seen to be effective on symptoms. (217) According to the American College Gastroenterology Clinic, fibre intake is an effective treatment in adults, but unwanted events such as bloating and cramps can occur, especially if gradual increases are not made in fibre intake, this could limit its use. Fibre has not only been proven to be beneficial in patients with slow-transit constipation, but is also useful in those with pelvic floor dysfunction. Although very rare, intestinal lower obstruction has been reported secondary to high fibre intake in elderly patients. (218)

✓ **Probiotics** are currently widely used as components of bio-yoghurts, as food supplements, and are medically prescribed. The faecal flora changes significantly with a decrease in the number of bifidobacteria. (219) However, whether this is a cause or an effect of constipation remains unclear. Studies have reported an increase in the concentration of SCFAs, a shortening of intestinal transit time and softening of stool with the use of probiotics in the elderly. (220) Probiotics can be evaluated in the treatment process as there are no side-effects nor any interaction with other drugs. However, significant benefits may not be seen in the complex clinical situation of geriatric constipation in large, randomised controlled studies.(219,220)

✓ **Chocolate** should be avoided as it can cause difficult defecation by increasing the viscosity of the stool. (221)

✓ **Fruits** are important in constipation diets. Fruits contain water, sorbitol, fructose, fibre and phytochemicals. Fruits considered to be beneficial in the treatment of constipation are those rich in fibre and include pears, grapes, plums and apples (unpeeled). Recent studies have also shown significant benefits of kiwi fruit, prunes, bananas and dates.(222)

**Kiwi,** in clinical studies involving adults, have shown to significantly increase the frequency of defecation, volume of stool, softness of bowel movements, and ease of defecation. The mechanisms suggested for this are: (222)

a) 100 gr kiwi includes 2–3 g dietary fibre, which plays a physicochemical role in constipation. (222)

b) Actinidin, which is a protease enzyme found in kiwi, stimulates upper GI tract motility. (222)

c) Kissper, which is a peptide in kiwi, is characterised by anion selectivity and ion channels. (222)

**Prunes** are beneficial for constipation as they include high levels of fibre (6.1 g/100 gr), fructose (fructant) and sorbitol (14.7 g/100 g). Large amounts of phenolic components (184 mg/100 gr), such as neochlorogenic and chlorogenic acids, may have a beneficial laxative effect. Prune juice contains less sorbitol and fibre than prunes. An experimental rat model demonstrated that prunes increased the frequency of defecation and contractions of the colon. (223)

**Dates** are one of the most popular fruits in Asia. There are several varieties of dates, which can be classified as soft dates with a low concentration of tannic acid and mature and dry dates with a high tannin content. Hardness of dates depends on the soluble tannins contained in the fruit. When the date ripens, soluble tannins become insoluble and this makes the fruit less sour. As the date grows in size, so does the total amount of tannin. Tannic acid decreases secretions in the small intestine and prevents peristalsis. (224)

**Banana:** 100 gr of ripe banana contains 100–250 mg tannin and has a starch content with high amylase resistance. Therefore, it can cause or exacerbate previously existing constipation. When the banana ripens, the amounts of tannin and amylase-resistant starch decrease, while soluble sugars increase. A 120 gr of ripe banana contains 3 gr fibre, mostly in the form of soluble fibre. It also contains amylase-resistant starch and tannins. (225)

**Mint oil** is an anti-spasmodic that inhibits calcium channels and leads to relaxation of the smooth muscles in the GI system. Different doses and treatment durations have been examined: 450–900 mg per day divided in 2–3 doses over 1–3 months.(226,227) The most commonly reported negative effect has been shown to be gastro-oesophageal reflux associated with partial relaxing effect of the oil on the oesophageal sphincter. (228)

✓ Foods containing oil and sugar, fast foods, fried foods and sweet drinks (especially carbonated drinks) should be avoided. The intake of foods that can cause constipation, such as white bread, potatoes, rice and fruit (bananas, stewed and grated apples) should be reduced. An increase in the intake of wholegrain bread, fruits and vegetables, such as pears, apples, pineapple, broccoli, carrots, and beans are useful in treatment of constipation. (229)

✓ Alcohol causes water extraction and hardening of stool. Fluid loss is increased. It is recommended that alcohol not be consumed, or its consumption should be reduced. (229)

✓ Of herbal teas available, green tea and fennel tea are helpful in increasing bowel movements; two to three cups per day can be consumed. Senna tea must be avoided as they can increase the risk of colon cancer.(229)

Exercise is also important in treatment of constipation. Starting with light physical activity, exercise is recommended with regular daily routines. The most appropriate times for bowel movements are after waking up and right after meals when normal colon motor activity is increased. (229)

## 2.2  A Sample Diet for the Prevention of Constipation

<u>Breakfast</u>

- 1 thin slice of Feta cheese
- Tomatoes, cucumber, pepper, parsley (with one teaspoon of olive oil)
- 2 prunes or dry apricots
- 1 thin slice of whole bread

<u>Snack</u>

- 1 kiwi fruit

<u>Lunch</u>

- 1 plate of vegetables or dry legume dish
- Salad
- Yoghurt (can be probiotic)
- 1 plate (5-6 tablespoons) wholegrain pasta or bulgur

<u>Snack</u>

- 1 glass of kefir or yoghurt (can be probiotic)

  Fruits (2 dried apricots)

<u>Dinner</u>

- 1 bowl of vegetable soup
- Salad
- Yoghurt (can be probiotic)

- Grilled fish + vegetables
- 1 thin slice of whole bread

**Snack**

- Fruit

## 2.3 Constipation in Children

Constipation is a widespread global problem not only for adults, but also for children.(230,231) Functional GI disorders are clinically present, characterised by impaired defecation without identifiable structural, anatomic or biochemical anomalies, and chronic recurrent abdominal pain and recurrent vomiting. (230,232) Functional constipation occurs at high rates in several geographies of the world. Childhood constipation is one of the most frequently seen disorders with a rate of 14 %. (232) FC shows variations in prevalence among geographic regions. While prevalence (including infants) varies between 10 % and 23 % in North and South America, it is between 0.7 % and 12 % in Europe (including only children) and 0.5 %–29.6 % (including infants–adolescents) in Asia.(232,233,234,235) Prevalence varies according to age groups. The incidence of constipation is seen to peak at age 2–4 years, when toilet training starts. In a recent systematic review, the mean prevalence of constipation in children was reported to be 12 %. (232)In infants, the incidence of constipation has been shown to be 0.05 %–39.3 %. (237)In the adult population, constipation is more evident in females but there are no clear data related to gender differences in infants and adolescents.(233,234,235,236,238) Major differences reported in the prevalence of childhood constipation may be due to several factors including methodology, variance in age groups and different definitions. (239)Constipation in children is generally functional or idiopathic and is associated with behavioural attitude following painful or unpleasant defecation.(237,240,241)

Although the pathophysiology of FC in children is unclear, it is multifactorial. If there is no underlying congenital cause, constipation is defined as FC. Associated with an organic cause at the rate of 5 %, the etiology varies from Hirschsprung disease, anorectal malformations, neuromuscular disease, and metabolic events to endocrine disorders. The most common mechanism for the development of FC, especially in young children, is generally the behaviour of retaining stools starting after a painful or frightening bowel movement. Rapidly changing sociocultural and political factors, such as urbanisation, increased psychological stress, inadequate parenting skills, civil unrest and maltreatment are major reasons for development of constipation in many children. (232)

The stools remain in the rectum, the rectal mucosa reabsorbs water from the retained stools, which become more difficult to evacuate.(242) In a subgroup of children, FC can be due to slow transit. The interstitial cells of Cajal play an important role in the motility of the gut. These cells can be regarded as pacemakers that generate peristalsis in the gut. Many publications report consistent histological findings in children with all forms of constipation of a low number of interstitial cells of Cajal, although the normal number of interstitial cells of Cajal in healthy children remains unclear. (243)

### 2.3.1 The Rome III Criteria for the Diagnosis of Functional Constipation in Children – For Infants and Children in the 0–4 Years Age Group

Presence of at least two of the following symptoms/habits for at least a duration of one month:(244)

- Defecation twice a week or less often,
- Faecal incontinence at least once a week after completing toilet training,
- A history of excessive stool accumulation,
- A history of painful and hard defecation,
- The presence of a large faecal mass in the rectum,
- A history of large diameter stool that can block the toilet.

### 2.3.2 For Children in the 4–18 Years Age Group

Presence of at least two of the following symptoms/habits for at least a duration of one month: (244)

- Defecation twice a week or less often,
- Faecal incontinence at least once a week,
- "Retentive posture" or a history of excessive voluntary stool retention,

- A history of painful and hard defecation,
- The presence of a large faecal mass in the rectum,
- A history of large diameter stool that can block the toilet.

The recently created Rome IV criteria were revised for children aged 0–4 years. Children that have not been toilet trained do not need to fulfil the two additional criteria for a diagnosis of FC. The excluded criteria are faecal incontinence at least once a week and large diameter stool that can block the toilet. The first criteria are not valid for this age group, but it is clear that other measures are also excluded as stool retention cannot be considered if toilet training has not been provided. Later, duration of symptoms can be shortened from 2 months to 1 month for ages 4 years to adolescence. (245)

### 2.3.3  Rome IV Criteria

Defined with the presence of two or more of the following symptoms/habits for at least one month: (246)

- Defecation ≤ twice a week,
- Excessive retention of stools,
- Painful or difficult bowel movements,
- Presence of a large faecal mass in the rectum,
- Large diameter and volume of stools,
- After the completion of toilet training, stool retention more than once a week.

Despite the recommendation of the Rome IV criteria as the new gold standard, they must be evaluated, just as all other definitions. The Rome criteria are suitable for the selection of FC patients at a comparable level, especially for clinical studies, but may be of less benefit for diagnosis in clinical practice. From a current perspective, there is a need for new studies to determine the value of the Rome criteria in the diagnosis of FC. (245)

### 2.3.4  Known Risk Factors for Childhood Constipation (247)

✓ Psychological stress
✓ Home related issues

✓ School related issues
✓ Siblings with health problems
✓ Lower social class
✓ Living away from parents
✓ Poor parenting skills
✓ Dietary problems
✓ Cow milk proteins
✓ Not eating meals with parents regularly
✓ Eating snack food
✓ Childhood obesity
✓ Maltreatment of the child
✓ Physical abuse
✓ Sexual abuse
✓ Emotional abuse
✓ Civil conflict (exposure to war)

• **Stress**

Psychological stress is a reason for FC development in children. In a school-based study in Sri Lanka, psychological stress related to home or school was noticeably related to FC in children. (248) Inan et al. reported that physical or psychological trauma, siblings with health problems, and other personal health problems led to development of FC. In such conditions, where parents have to leave the child in care of grandparents, a home nanny or at a day care centre are known to have a negative effect on normal bowel habits and healthy toilet routines. (249) In addition, factors such as a long times spent doing homework for school and lack of sleep are potential risk factors for development of FC in children.(250) Civil conflict, internal political unrest and war are also known to be associated with FGDs. Although exact mechanism is not fully understood, changes in stress mediators of both the brain-intestine axis and the hypothalamopituitary-adrenal axis contribute to the development of abnormal colon and rectal functions, which lead to development of IBS. (251,252,253)

• **Parenting styles**

A study in Holland showed that e children of large families with high autonomy points had a significantly lower frequency of defecation. (254)

- **Abuse**

Maltreatment of children is another social welfare problem worldwide. In developed countries, it has been reported that children experience physical abuse at the rate of 4 %–16 %, sexual abuse at 5 %–10 % and are psychologically deprived or neglected at the rate of 10 %. (255)In developing countries, these rates are worse at 83 % of children experiencing psychological abuse and 64 % physical abuse.(256) A study in Sri Lanka demonstrated a correlation between physical, psychological or sexual abuse and constipation. Furthermore, children with constipation and a history of abuse had more severe intestinal symptoms and higher somatisation scores. (257) Maltreatment of a child leads to severe psychological stress, which may cause permanent changes in GI motility, visceral sensitivity, changes in autonomic functions, and hypothalamopituitary-adrenal dysfunction. (258)

- **Familial Predisposition**

A study in Iran reported that there was a higher tendency for mothers of children with constipation to have similar problems. (259) Another study also found a higher tendency for children with constipation to have siblings or parents also suffering from constipation. However, to date there have been no correlating studies or direct gene sequence studies that have identified any specific gene mutation. (261)

- **Psychological Comorbidities**

The role of psychological and emotional components in the etiology of FC is a matter of debate. While some researchers advocate that emotional problems result from FC, others believe they play an important role in the etiology. In a study in Holland using a child behaviour checklist, it was shown that these children have a series of abnormal behaviour characteristics. (262) Other studies have also demonstrated that these children have abnormal personality characteristics and have a higher tendency for anxiety disorders. (263,264) These factors can have a negative effect on social and family life. It has been shown that the total medical costs of anxiety are 184 % more than for depression, causing an increase of 348 % in costs per patient and an increase of 97 % in total medical costs.(265) Therefore, comorbid psychiatric disorders lead to higher medical costs and increased public health issues. However, in majority of the patients, these behavioural problems are mild and can be resolved following regular treatment. (262)

**Family** Some researchers believe that a mild disease such as constipation does not affect the family. However, in a study of children with constipation and their families, conducted in Milwaukee, USA, parental feelings were stated as "angry, worried, sad, irritable, and ashamed". (266) Data from China related to the effect on the family of chronic constipation have shown that the parents of children with FC have a poor HRQoL and there is a significant negative effect on communication with parents, family functioning, daily activity in the family and relationships as well. Reports reveal that the parents of children with FC were constantly worried about their children. (267)

- **Obesity**

Obesity is widespread throughout the world, and data have shown that it is at a level of concern. (268) Some studies have shown that FC is related to obesity. In Paediatric Gastroenterology Clinics, obesity has been found to be a risk factor for the development of FC. (269) In a general paediatric clinical study performed in the USA, it was reported that obese children have a higher predisposition for FC; while a study in Holland showed that the prevalence of FC was found to be higher in morbidly obese children. (270) However, in a recent population-based study in Colombia, no such relationship was found. (271)

- **Fast-food and Physical Activity**

Fast-food consumption has become an increasingly widespread practice. Studies have shown that the consumption of "junk food" is related to constipation. In a study in China, it was reported that children and adolescents who consumed fast-food were at much higher risk for FGDs. Previous studies have also shown that lack of physical exercise is another risk factor for low frequency of defecation and FC. (248,272,273)

- **Dietary Factors**

Diet and nutritional habits are of great importance, both in the formation of constipation and its treatment. Dietary factors are known to play a significant role in the development of FC in children. (274,250,275,277) The inclusion of important amounts of fibre (age [years]+ 5g/day) is recommended in the diet of children. Several studies have shown that FC development is related to a low-fibre diet. The data in respect to an association between cow milk protein allergy and FC development are inconsistent.(276) Iacono et al. reported that after removing cow milk from the diet, 68 % of children with FC recovered. (277) When milk was given again in the diet, all the children developed the symptoms of FC. Similarly, Daher et al. showed a relationship between constipation and cow milk protein allergy. However, more recent data are in contrast to those findings. The relationship between cow milk and FC was evaluated in a study in Italy. The results showed a similar prevalence of atopy in the FC children and the control group, reporting that an elimination diet was of no benefit to children with FC. Restriction of cow milk is a widespread practice for children with FC. However, cow milk is generally the source of protein and restricting it without proper evidence could deprive the balanced diet of a child.

Most cases of chronic constipation in young children can be explained by functional changes secondary to a low-fibre diet and early withdrawal of milk.

Another risk factor for constipation is low fluid intake. (278)

## 2.3.5 Treatment

There are pharmacological and non-pharmacological treatment methods for the management of functional constipation in children. (279)

| Pharmacological Methods | Non-pharmacological methods |
|---|---|
| • Osmotic laxatives (magnesium hydroxide, magnesium sulphate, lactic, lactulose, glycerine suppositories) | • Education |
| | • Behavioural therapy |
| | • Biofeedback |
| • Stimulants (bisacodyl, Indian oil) | • High-fibre diet |
| • Softeners (sodium, liquid paraffin) | • Increased fluid intake |
| • Mass producing substances (methylcellulose, dietary fibre, psillium) | • Exercise |
| | • Psychotherapy |
| • Serotonin receptor agonists (Tegaserod) | |
| • Spasmolytics (Trimebutine) | |
| • Probiotics (conflicting data) | |

Functional constipation treatment requires parental education, behavioural interventions, precautions to be taken that provide bowel movements at normal intervals with good excretion, close follow-ups, adjustment of drugs and necessary evaluations. (280,281,282)

### 2.3.6 Education and Behavioural Changes

Behavioural training helps the child to understand that the defecation process is a routine activity and encourages a child not to retain stools. This method increases awareness and decreases the fear of defecation. Strategies appropriate to the development of the child are used in behavioural training, such as pictures, stories and games. The strategies are used to teach the correct position, holding breath and relaxation techniques. (279)

The first stage of treatment is education. Toilet training is one of the significant factors in the treatment process. This means a regular training process for the child to use a toilet/potty. There is a natural reflex mechanism (gastrochoal, gastrocolic and duodenic reflexes) which stimulates defecation working approximately 20-30 min after the main meal. Regular toileting after meals (5-10 min) combined with a reward system is generally helpful for behavioural change. Despite the importance of behavioural changes and education, with the exception of rare cases of underlying behavioural problems, intense behavioural therapy does not contribute to the success of treatment. (283) Some studies have shown that biological feedback is not effective for children with FC. (280,284)

### 2.3.7 Education of Parents

Family members must be educated on the additional advantages of treatment and the need to avoid mistakes throughout the whole treatment process. Parents should be encouraged to display a positive and supportive attitude throughout the treatment. Following diets, constructive and supportive behaviour should be shown to the child. (279)

### 2.3.8 Precautions to be Taken that Provide Bowel Movements at Normal Intervals with Good Evacuation (Precautions against Impaction) and Drug Therapy

When there is faecal impaction, prevention with oral and rectal drugs is necessary before starting treatment. Although oral drugs are less invasive, they require more patient collaboration and ameliorate symptoms more slowly. There are several therapies available.(280,285,286) The emergence of polyethylene glycol-based solutions (PEG) (Miralax) changed the initial approach to children with constipation as they are non-invasive, effective, easy-to-apply and well-tolerated. (287) The use of NASPGHAN/ESPGHAN, polyethylene glycol (PEG) (0.2–0.8 gr/kg) with or without electrolytes, is recommended.

Although there is some evidence of PEG support as the first stage of treatment, general data has not shown any clear advantage of laxatives, which are usually used as medical treatment. (288) There may be side-effects of laxatives, depending on the dose. Lactulose, sorbitol, milk of magnesia and mineral oil show an equal level of effect in children. The taste of milk of magnesia and mineral oil is not pleasant, and mineral oil is contra-indicated in infants because of the risk of lipoid pneumonia. The laxative that was widely used in children until the advent of PEG was lactulose.(289) In a study by Loening-Baucke, low-volume PEG (0.5–1 gr/kg/day) not containing electrolytes was shown to be as effective as milk of magnesia.(290) A meta-analysis of five randomised, controlled studies, including 519 children, compared low-volume PEG with lactulose in the treatment of paediatric FC, with PEG observed to have equivalent tolerability to lactulose, and was more effective with fewer side-effects, such as bloating and pain.(291) In long-term use, the efficacy of lactulose is mainly associated with change in the gut flora. The laxative dose should be adjusted according to the type of stool.(292)

## 2.3.9 Laxatives – Dosages and Side-Effects (289)

| Drugs | Dose | Side-effects |
|---|---|---|
| Lactulose | 1–2 g/kg, 1–2 dose | Bloating, abdominal cramps |
| Sorbitol | 1–3 mL/kg/day, 1–2 dose | Bloating, abdominal cramps |
| Milk of Magnesia | 1–3 mL/kg/day, 1–2 dose | Overuse leads to hypocalcaemia, hypermagnesemia, hypophosphatemia |
| PEG to remove impaction | 25 mL/kg/hour(R/T) or 1-1.5 g/kg 3-6 days | Bloating, cramps, nausea and vomiting |
| PEG to maintain status-quo | 5–10 mL/kg/day or 0.4 to 0.8 g/kg/day | Bloating, cramps, nausea and vomiting |
| Mineral oil to remove impaction | 15–30 mL/ age in years (max 240mL) | Lipoid pneumonia, inhibition of the absorption of fat-soluble vitamins |

| Drugs | Dose | Side-effects |
| --- | --- | --- |
| Mineral oil to maintain status-quo | 1–3 mL / kg / day | Lipoid pneumonia, inhibition of the absorption of fat-soluble vitamins |
| Senna | 2–6 years: 2.5–7.5 mL/day (8.8 mg/5mL) 6-12 years: 5-15 mL/day | Melanosis coli, hepatitis, hypertrophy |
| Bisacodyl | 0.5–1 suppository (10 mg)1-3 nail /dose (5 mg) | Abdominal pain, diarrhoea, hypokalaemia |

## 2.4 Diet Treatment

Changing the diet and nutritional habits is part of effective treatment of FC. Nutritional habits and a balanced diet for the prevention and treatment of constipation should include the following principles.(279)

- **Fibre-rich foods**

Fibre stimulates gastrointestinal peristalsis, softens stool by absorbing water and increases colon sensitivity to mechanical stimuli. Daily consumption of fibre-rich foods at specific times makes positive effects in the management of constipation.

The daily dose can be calculated according to the following formula:

Age (years)+5= fibre (g) / day

The fibre dosage must be calculated separately for each patient and should be gradually increased by quarter teaspoon measures until the recommended daily fibre dose is reached and/or there is faecal softening. If fibre intake is stopped, all beneficial effects are lost. (293)

- **Fluid intake**

The recommendations of Holiday and Segar are among the most useful methods for calculating the total fluid intake (as ml) for children.

For children with body weight of 1–10 kg: 100ml/kg

For children with body weight of 11–20 kg:1000ml + 50 ml / kg for every 10kg body weight

For children with body weight >20kg: 1500 ml + 20ml for every kg over 20 kg.

Daily milk consumption should be limited to 230–350 ml, depending on the age of the child. Fruit juice should be limited to 120 ml/day; fresh and dry fruit (apple and prunes) and vegetables should be used instead. The remaining fluid requirement should be met with only water intake. (294)

- **Avoidance of foods containing fat and sugar, fast-foods, fried foods and sweet drinks (especially carbonated drinks)**

The intake of foods that can cause constipation, such as white bread, potatoes, rice and fruit (bananas, stewed and grated apples) should be reduced. An increase in the intake of wholegrain bread, fruits and vegetables (pears, apples, pineapple, broccoli, carrots, beans) is useful in the treatment of constipation. (295)

- **Use of herbs and spices**

Dill tea, chamomile tea, olive oil (added to soup), and honey with water in the mornings are useful in the treatment of constipation for children over 2 years of age. (295)

- **Physical Activity**

In addition to the organisation of a nutritional plan, getting the habit of regular physical activity is important in the treatment of constipation. There should be a maximum of 2 hours per day of regular physical activity, including daily outdoor activity, with a reduction of screen time (television, computer). (295)

- **Probiotics Use**

There is a conflicting evidence about the beneficial effects of probiotics for children with constipation. Some researchers have confirmed that there are positive effects, drawing attention to the effects on motor activity of the GI system, with a reduction in saccharide bacteria such as bifidobacteria and lactobacillus, fermented fibres in SCFAs, and intestinal pH, resulting in increased intestinal motility. On the basis of this hypothesis, the use of probiotics has been considered useful in the treatment of constipation, especially with effects on lactobacillus and bifidobacteria. However, others have reported that probiotics are of no benefit in the treatment of FC. To reach a consensus on this point, there is a need for further large-scale, double-blind, randomised, placebo-controlled studies.(297)

# List of Figures

# List of Tables

# Bibliography

1 Mayer EA. Clinical practice. Irritable bowel syndrome. N Engl J Med 2008;358:1692–1699.

2 Drossman DA, Camilleri M, Mayer E, Whitehead WE. AGA technical review on irritable bowel syndrome. Gastroenterology 2002;123:21082131.

3 Aleksandrova K, Mosquera B. R, Hernandez V. Diet, Gut Microbiome and epigenetics: emerging links with inflammatory bowel diseases and prospects for management and prevention. Nutrients. 2017;9: 962. doi:10.3390/nu9090962.

4 Molodecky, N.A.; Soon, I.S.; Rabi, D.M.; Ghali, W.A.; Ferris, M.; Chernoff, G.; Benchimol, E.I.; Panaccione, R.; Ghosh, S.; Barkema, H.W.; et al. Increasing incidence and prevalence of the inflammatory bowel diseases with time, based on systematic review. Gastroenterology 2012, 142, 46–54. [CrossRef] [PubMed]

5 Lee,D.;Albenberg, L.;Compher, C.;Baldassano, R.;Piccoli, D.;Lewis, J.D.;Wu, G.D. Diet in the pathogenesis and treatment of inflammatory bowel diseases. Gastroenterology 2015, 148, 1087–1106. [CrossRef] [PubMed] 8. Lovasz, B.D.; Golovics, P.A.; Vegh,Z.; Lakatos,P.L. New trends in inflammatory bowel disease epidemiology and disease course in eastern europe. Dig. Liver Dis. 2013, 45, 269–276. [CrossRef] [PubMed]

6 Lophaven, S.N.; Lynge, E.; Burisch, J. The incidence of inflammatory bowel disease in Denmark 1980–2013: A nationwide cohort study. Aliment. Pharmacol. Ther. 2017, 45, 961–972. [CrossRef] [PubMed]

7 Simrén M, Törnblom H, Palsson OS, van Tilburg MAL, Van Oudenhove L, Tack J, Whitehead WE. Visceral hypersensitivity is associated with GI symptom severity in functional GI disorders: consistent findings from five different patient cohorts. Gut. 2017; pii: gutjnl-2016-312361 [PMID: 28104632 DOI: 10.1136/ gutjnl-2016-312361]

8 Ford AC, Talley NJ. Mucosal inflammation as a potential etiological factor in irritable bowel syndrome: a systematic review. J Gastroenterol 2011; 46: 421–431 [PMID: 21331765 DOI: 10.1007/ s00535-011-0379-9]

9    Ikechi R, Fischer B.D, DeSipio J, and Phadtare S. Irritable
     Bowel Syndrome: clinical manifestations, dietary influences,
     and management. Healthcare 2017; 5 (21): 1–14. doi:10.3390/
     healthcare5020021.

10   Desipio,J.; Friedenberg, F.K.; Korimilli, A.; Richter, J.E.; Parkman,
     H.P.; Fisher, R.S. High-resolution solid-state manometry of the antro
     pyloro duodenal region. Neurogastroenterol. Motil. 2007, 19,
     188–195. [CrossRef] [PubMed]

11   Malik, A.; Lukaszewski, K.; Caroline, D.; Parkman, H. A
     retrospective review of enteroclysis in patients with obscure
     gastrointestinal bleeding and chronic abdominal pain of undetermined
     etiology. Dig. Dis. Sci. 2005, 50, 649–655. [CrossRef] [PubMed]

12   Barbara G, Feinle-Bisset C, Ghoshal UC, Quigley EM, Santos J,
     Vanner S, et al. The intestinal microenvironment and functional
     gastrointestinal disorders. Gastroenterology. 2016;150(6):1305–18.

13   Gazouli M, Wouters MM, Kapur-Pojskic ´ L, Bengtson M-B,
     Friedman E, Nikcĕvic ´ G, et al. Lessons learned—resolving the
     enigma of genetic factors in IBS. Nat Rev Gastroenterol Hepatol.
     2016;13(2):77.

14   Enck P, Aziz Q, Barbara G, Farmer AD, Fukudo S, Mayer EA, et al.
     Irritable bowel syndrome. Nat Rev Dis Primer. 2016;2:16014.

15   Ford AC, Lacy BE, Talley NJ. Irritable bowel syndrome. N Engl J
     Med. 2017;376:2566–78.

16   Kostic, A.D.; Xavier, R.J.; Gevers, D. The microbiome in
     inflammatory bowel disease: Current status and the future ahead.
     Gastroenterology 2014, 146, 1489–1499. [CrossRef] [PubMed]

17   Prosberg, M.; Bendtsen, F.; Vind, I.; Petersen, A.M.; Gluud, L.L. The
     association between the gut microbiota and the inflammatory bowel
     disease activity: A systematic review and meta-analysis. Scand. J.
     Gastroenterol. 2016, 51, 1407–1415. [CrossRef] [PubMed]

18   Wills, E.S.; Jonkers, D.M.A.E.; Savelkoul, P.H.; Masclee, A.A.; Pierik,
     M.J.; Penders, J. Fecal microbial composition of ulcerative colitis and
     Crohn's disease patients in remission and subsequent exacerbation.
     PLoS ONE 2014, 9, e90981. [CrossRef] [PubMed]

19   Varela, E.; Manichanh, C.; Gallart, M.; Torrejón, A.; Borruel,
     N.; Casellas, F.; Guarner, F.; Antolin, M. Colonisation by

Faecalibacterium prausnitzii and maintenance of clinical remission in patients with ulcerative colitis. Aliment. Pharmacol. Ther. 2013, 38, 151–161. [CrossRef] [PubMed]

20 Dominguez- Bello, M.G.; Costello, E.K.; Contreras, M.; Magris, M.; Hidalgo, G.; Fierer, N.; Knight, R. Delivery mode shapes the acquisition and structure of the initial microbiota across multiple body habitats in newborns. Proc. Natl. Acad. Sci. USA 2010, 107, 11971–11975. [CrossRef] [PubMed]

21 Scarpa, M.; Stylianou, E. Epigenetics: Concepts and relevance to IBD pathogenesis. Inflamm. BowelDis. 2012, 18, 1982–1996. [CrossRef] [PubMed]

22 Ventham, N.T.; Kennedy, N.A.; Nimmo, E.R.; Satsangi, J. Beyond gene discovery in inflammatory bowel disease: The emerging role of epigenetics. Gastroenterology 2013, 145, 293–308. [CrossRef] [PubMed]

23 Anderson, C.A.; Boucher, G.; Lees, C.W.; Franke, A.; D'Amato, M.; Taylor, K.D.; Lee, J.C.; Goyette, P.; Imielinski, M.; Latiano, A.; et al. Meta-analysis identifies 29 additional ulcerative colitis risk loci, increasing the number of confirmed associations to 47. Nat. Genet. 2011, 43, 246–252. [CrossRef] [PubMed]

24 Beaudet, A.L. Epigenetics and complex human disease: Is there a role in IBD? J. Pediatr. Gastroenterol. Nutr. 2008, 46, E2. [PubMed]

25 Chapman, C.G.; Pekow, J. The emerging role of mirnas in inflammatory bowel disease: A review. Ther. Adv. Gastroenterol. 2015, 8, 4–22. [CrossRef] [PubMed]

26 Kalla, R.; Ventham, N.T.; Kennedy, N.A.; Quintana, J.F.; Nimmo, E.R.; Buck, A.H.; Satsangi, J. MicroRNAs: New players in IBD. Gut 2015, 64, 504–517. [CrossRef] [PubMed]

27 Harris, R.A.; Nagy-Szakal, D.; Pedersen, N.; Opekun, A.; Bronsky, J.; Munkholm, P.; Jespersgaard, C.; Andersen, P.; Melegh, B.; Ferry, G.; et al. Genome-wide peripheral blood leukocyte DNA methylation microarrays identified a single association with inflammatory bowel diseases. Inflamm. Bowel Dis. 2012, 18, 2334–2341. [CrossRef] [PubMed]

28 Oświęcimska J, Szymlak A, Roczniak W, Girczys-Połedniok K, Kwiecień J. New insights into the pathogenesis and treatment of

irritable bowel syndrome. Adv Med Sci 2017; 62: 17–30 [PMID: 28135659 DOI: 10.1016/j.advms.2016.11.001]

29   Gibson PR. Food intolerance in functional bowel disorders. J Gastroenterol Hepatol 2011; 26 Suppl 3: 128–131 [PMID: 21443725 DOI: 10.1111/j.1440-1746.2011.06650.x]

30   Cuomo R, Andreozzi P, Zito FP, Passananti V, De Carlo G, Sarnelli G. Irritable bowel syndrome and food interaction. World J Gastroenterol 2014; 20: 8837–8845 [PMID: 25083057 DOI: 10.3748/wjg.v20. i27.8837]

31   Böhn L, Störsrud S, Törnblom H, Bengtsson U, Simrén M. Self-reported food-related gastrointestinal symptoms in IBS are common and associated with more severe symptoms and reduced quality of life. Am J Gastroenterol 2013; 108: 634–641 [PMID: 23644955 DOI: 10.1038/ajg.2013.105]

32   Monsbakken KW, Vandvik PO, Farup PG. Perceived food intolerance in subjects with irritable bowel syndrome-- etiology, prevalence and consequences. Eur J Clin Nutr 2006; 60: 667–672 [PMID: 16391571 DOI: 10.1038/sj.ejcn.1602367]

33   Ostgaard H, Hausken T, Gundersen D, El-Salhy M. Diet and effects of diet management on quality of life and symptoms in patients with irritable bowel syndrome. Mol Med Rep 2012; 5: 1382–1390 [PMID: 22446969 DOI: 10.3892/mmr.2012.843]

34   McKenzie YA, Bowyer RK, Leach H, Gulia P, Horobin J, O' Sullivan NA, Pettitt C, Reeves LB, Seamark L, Williams M, Thompson J, Lomer MC. British Dietetic Association systematic review and evidence-based practice guidelines for the dietary management of irritable bowel syndrome in adults (2016 update). J Hum Nutr Diet 2016; 29: 549–575 [PMID: 27272325 DOI: 10.1111/jhn.12385]

35   National Institute for Health and Clinical Excellence. Irritable bowel syndrome in adults: diagnosis and management. Clinical Guideline [CG61]. Published: February 2008. Last updated: February 2015. Cited 2017-01-03. Available from: URL: https:// www.nice.org.uk/ guidance/cg61/resources/irritable-bowelsyndrome-in-adults-diagnosis-and-management-975562917829

36   Miwa H. Life style in persons with functional gastrointestinal disorders--large-scale internet survey of lifestyle in Japan.

Neurogastroenterol Motil 2012; 24: 464–471, e217 [PMID: 22292849 DOI: 10.1111/j.1365-2982.2011.01872.x]

37  Guo YB, Zhuang KM, Kuang L, Zhan Q, Wang XF, Liu SD. Association between Diet and Lifestyle Habits and Irritable Bowel Syndrome: A Case-Control Study. Gut Liver 2015; 9: 649–656 [PMID: 25266811 DOI: 10.5009/gnl13437]

38  Crowell MD, Cheskin LJ, Musial F. Prevalence of gastrointestinal symptoms in obese and normal weight binge eaters. Am J Gastroenterol 1994; 89: 387–391 [PMID: 8122651]

39  Heizer WD, Southern S, McGovern S. The role of diet in symptoms of irritable bowel syndrome in adults: a narrative review. J Am Diet Assoc 2009; 109: 1204–1214 [PMID: 19559137 DOI: 10.1016/j. jada.2009.04.012]

40  Hayes P, Corish C, O'Mahony E, Quigley EM. A dietary survey of patients with irritable bowel syndrome. J Hum Nutr Diet 2014; 27 Suppl 2: 36–47 [PMID: 23659729 DOI: 10.1111/jhn.12114]

41  Simrén M, Månsson A, Langkilde AM, Svedlund J, Abrahamsson H, Bengtsson U, Björnsson ES. Food-related gastrointestinal symptoms in the irritable bowel syndrome. Digestion 2001; 63: 108–115 [PMID: 11244249]

42  Esmaillzadeh A, Keshteli AH, Hajishafiee M, Feizi A, FeinleBisset C, Adibi P. Consumption of spicy foods and the prevalence of irritable bowel syndrome. World J Gastroenterol 2013; 19: 6465–6471 [PMID: 24151366 DOI: 10.3748/wjg.v19.i38.6465]

43  Gonlachanvit S, Fongkam P, Wittayalertpanya S, Kullavanijaya P. Red chili induces rectal hypersensitivity in healthy humans: possible role of 5HT-3 receptors on capsaicin-sensitive visceral nociceptive pathways. Aliment Pharmacol Ther 2007; 26: 617–625 [PMID: 17661765 DOI: 10.1111/j.1365-2036.2007.03396.x]

44  Hammer J, Vogelsang H. Characterization of sensations induced by capsaicin in the upper gastrointestinal tract. Neurogastroenterol Motil 2007; 19: 279–287 [PMID: 17391244 DOI: 10.1111/ j.1365-2982.2007.00900.x]

45  Chan CL, Facer P, Davis JB, Smith GD, Egerton J, Bountra C, Williams NS, Anand P. Sensory fibres expressing capsaicin receptor TRPV1 in patients with rectal hypersensitivity and faecal urgency. Lancet 2003; 361: 385–391 [PMID: 12573376]

46  Akbar A, Yiangou Y, Facer P, Walters JR, Anand P, Ghosh S.
    Increased capsaicin receptor TRPV1-expressing sensory fibres in
    irritable bowel syndrome and their correlation with abdominal
    pain. Gut 2008; 57: 923–929 [PMID: 18252749 DOI: 10.1136/
    gut.2007.138982]

47  Agarwal MK, Bhatia SJ, Desai SA, Bhure U, Melgiri S. Effect of red
    chillies on small bowel and colonic transit and rectal sensitivity in
    men with irritable bowel syndrome. Indian J Gastroenterol 2002; 21:
    179–182 [PMID: 12416746]

48  Jowett SL, Seal CJ, Pearce MS, Phillips E, Gregory W, Barton JR,
    Welfare MR. Influence of dietary factors on the clinical course of
    ulcerative colitis: a prospective cohort study. Gut 2004; 53: 1479–
    1484 [PMID: 15361498 DOI: 10.1136/gut.2003.024828]

49  Uchiyama K, Nakamura M, Odahara S, Koido S, Katahira K,
    Shiraishi H, Ohkusa T, Fujise K, Tajiri H. N-3 polyunsaturated fatty
    acid diet therapy for patients with inflammatory bowel disease.
    Inflamm Bowel Dis 2010; 16: 1696–1707 [PMID: 20222122 DOI:
    10.1002/ibd.21251]

50  Faresjö A, Johansson S, Faresjö T, Roos S, Hallert C. Sex differences
    in dietary coping with gastrointestinal symptoms. Eur J Gastroenterol
    Hepatol 2010; 22: 327–333 [PMID: 19550348 DOI: 10.1097/
    MEG.0b013e32832b9c53]

51  Hayes P, Corish C, O'Mahony E, Quigley EM. A dietary survey of
    patients with irritable bowel syndrome. J Hum Nutr Diet 2014; 27
    Suppl 2: 36–47 [PMID: 23659729 DOI: 10.1111/jhn.12114]

52  Halpert A, Dalton CB, Palsson O, Morris C, Hu Y, Bangdiwala
    S, Hankins J, Norton N, Drossman D. What patients know
    about irritable bowel syndrome (IBS) and what they would like
    to know. National Survey on Patient Educational Needs in IBS
    and development and validation of the Patient Educational Needs
    Questionnaire (PEQ). Am J Gastroenterol 2007; 102: 1972–1982

53  Passos MC, Serra J, Azpiroz F, Tremolaterra F, Malagelada JR.
    Impaired reflex control of intestinal gas transit in patients with
    abdominal bloating. Gut 2005; 54: 344–348 [PMID: 15710981 DOI:
    10.1136/gut.2003.038158]

54  Salvioli B, Serra J, Azpiroz F, Malagelada JR. Impaired small
    bowel gas propulsion in patients with bloating during intestinal

lipid infusion. Am J Gastroenterol 2006; 101: 1853–1857 [PMID: 16817837 DOI: 10.1111/j.1572-0241.2006.00702.x]

55   Caldarella MP, Milano A, Laterza F, Sacco F, Balatsinou C, Lapenna D, Pierdomenico SD, Cuccurullo F, Neri M. Visceral sensitivity and symptoms in patients with constipation- or diarrhea predominant irritable bowel syndrome (IBS): effect of a low-fat intraduodenal infusion. Am J Gastroenterol 2005; 100: 383–389 [PMID: 15667496 DOI: 10.1111/j.1572-0241.2005.40100.x]

56   Simrén M, Abrahamsson H, Björnsson ES. Lipid-induced colonic hypersensitivity in the irritable bowel syndrome: the role of bowel habit, sex, and psychologic factors. Clin Gastroenterol Hepatol 2007; 5: 201–208 [PMID: 17174611 DOI: 10.1016/ j.cgh.2006.09.032]

57   Jarrett M, Heitkemper MM, Bond EF, Georges J. Comparison of diet composition in women with and without functional bowel disorder. Gastroenterol Nurs 1994; 16: 253–258 [PMID: 8075160]

58   Feinle-Bisset C, Azpiroz F. Dietary lipids and functional gastrointestinal disorders. Am J Gastroenterol 2013; 108: 737–747 [PMID: 23567355 DOI: 10.1038/ajg.2013.76]

59   Michalak A, Mosińska P, Fichna J. Polyunsaturated Fatty Acids and Their Derivatives: Therapeutic Value for Inflammatory, Functional Gastrointestinal Disorders, and Colorectal Cancer. Front Pharmacol 2016; 7: 459 [PMID: 27990120 DOI: 10.3389/ fphar.2016.00459]

60   Food and Agriculture Organisation (FAO), World Health Organisation (WHO). Fats and fatty acids in human nutrition. Report of an expert consultation. Food and Agriculture Organisation of the United Nations, Rome 2010. FAO Food and Nutrition Paper No. 91. Cited 2017-01-14. Available from: URL: http://www.fao.org/3/a-i1953e.pdf

61   Cuomo R, Andreozzi P, Zito FP, Passananti V, De Carlo G, Sarnelli G. Irritable bowel syndrome and food interaction. World J Gastroenterol 2014; 20: 8837–8845 [PMID: 25083057 DOI: 10.3748/wjg.v20. i27.8837]

62   Pohl D, Savarino E, Hersberger M, Behlis Z, Stutz B, Goetze O, Eckardstein AV, Fried M, Tutuian R. Excellent agreement between genetic and hydrogen breath tests for lactase deficiency and the role of extended symptom assessment. Br J Nutr 2010; 104: Cozma-Petruţ A et al. Dietary recommendations for IBS 3781 June 7, 2017|Volume

23|Issue 21|WJG |www.wjgnet.com 900–907 [PMID: 20398434 DOI: 10.1017/S0007114510001297]

63 Vernia P, Marinaro V, Argnani F, Di Camillo M, Caprilli R. Selfreported milk intolerance in irritable bowel syndrome: what should we believe? Clin Nutr 2004; 23: 996–1000 [PMID: 15380888 DOI: 10.1016/j.clnu.2003.12.005]

64 Yang J, Deng Y, Chu H, Cong Y, Zhao J, Pohl D, Misselwitz B, Fried M, Dai N, Fox M. Prevalence and presentation of lactose intolerance and effects on dairy product intake in healthy subjects and patients with irritable bowel syndrome. Clin Gastroenterol Hepatol 2013; 11: 262–268.e1 [PMID: 23246646 DOI: 10.1016/ j.cgh.2012.11.034]

65 Jianqin S, Leiming X, Lu X, Yelland GW, Ni J, Clarke AJ. Effects of milk containing only A2 beta casein versus milk containing both A1 and A2 beta casein proteins on gastrointestinal physiology, symptoms of discomfort, and cognitive behavior of people with self-reported intolerance to traditional cows' milk. Nutr J 2016; 15: 35 [PMID: 27039383 DOI: 10.1186/s12937-016-0147-z]

66 Saito YA, Locke GR, Weaver AL, Zinsmeister AR, Talley NJ. Diet and functional gastrointestinal disorders: a population-based casecontrol study. Am J Gastroenterol 2005; 100: 2743–2748 [PMID: 16393229 DOI: 10.1111/j.1572-0241.2005.00288.x]

67 Caldarella MP, Milano A, Laterza F, Sacco F, Balatsinou C, Lapenna D, Pierdomenico SD, Cuccurullo F, Neri M. Visceral sensitivity and symptoms in patients with constipation- or diarrheapredominant irritable bowel syndrome (IBS): effect of a low-fat intraduodenal infusion. Am J Gastroenterol 2005; 100: 383–389 [PMID: 15667496 DOI: 10.1111/j.1572-0241.2005.40100.x]

68 Halder SL, Locke GR, Schleck CD, Zinsmeister AR, Talley NJ. Influence of alcohol consumption on IBS and dyspepsia. Neurogastroenterol Motil 2006; 18: 1001–1008 [PMID: 17040411 Cozma-Petruţ A et al . Dietary recommendations for IBS

69 Moayyedi P, Quigley EM, Lacy BE, Lembo AJ, Saito YA, Schiller LR, Soffer EE, Spiegel BM, Ford AC. The effect of fiber supplementation on irritable bowel syndrome: a systematic review and meta-analysis. Am J Gastroenterol 2014; 109: 1367–1374 [PMID: 25070054 DOI: 10.1038/ajg.2014.195]

70 El-Salhy M, Gundersen D. Diet in irritable bowel syndrome. Nutr J 2015; 14: 36 [PMID: 25880820 DOI: 10.1186/ s12937-015-0022-3]

71  Capili B, Anastasi JK, Chang M. Addressing the Role of Food in
    Irritable Bowel Syndrome Symptom Management. J Nurse Pract 2016;
    12: 324–329 [PMID: 27429601 DOI: 10.1016/j.nurpra. 2015.12.007]

72  McRorie JW. Evidence-Based Approach to Fiber Supplements
    and Clinically Meaningful Health Benefits, Part 1: What to
    Look for and How to Recommend an Effective Fiber Therapy.
    Nutr Today 2015; 50: 82–89 [PMID: 25972618 DOI: 10.1097/
    NT.0000000000000082]

73  Ruepert L, Quartero AO, de Wit NJ, van der Heijden GJ, Rubin G,
    Muris JW. Bulking agents, antispasmodics and antidepressants for the
    treatment of irritable bowel syndrome. Cochrane Database Syst Rev
    2011; (8): CD003460 [PMID: 21833945 DOI: 10.1002/14651858.
    CD003460.pub3]

74  Eswaran S, Tack J, Chey WD. Food: the forgotten factor in the
    irritable bowel syndrome. Gastroenterol Clin North Am 2011; 40:
    141–162 [PMID: 21333905 DOI: 10.1016/j.gtc.2010.12.012]

75  Rao SS, Welcher K, Zimmerman B, Stumbo P. Is coffee a colonic
    stimulant? Eur J Gastroenterol Hepatol 1998; 10: 113–118 [PMID:
    9581985]

76  Simrén M, Månsson A, Langkilde AM, Svedlund J, Abrahamsson H,
    Bengtsson U, Björnsson ES. Food-related gastrointestinal symptoms
    in the irritable bowel syndrome. Digestion 2001; 63: 108–115
    [PMID: 11244249]

77  Reding KW, Cain KC, Jarrett ME, Eugenio MD, Heitkemper
    MM. Relationship between patterns of alcohol consumption and
    gastrointestinal symptoms among patients with irritable bowel
    syndrome. Am J Gastroenterol 2013; 108: 270–276 [PMID:
    23295280 DOI: 10.1038/ajg.2012.414]

78  McKenzie YA, Reeves LB, Williams M. Food fact sheet. Irritable
    bowel syndrome and diet. Published: January 2016. Cited 2017-
    01-05. Available from: URL: https://www.bda.uk.com/ foodfacts/
    IBSfoodfacts.pdf

79  U.S. Department of Health and Human Services and U.S. Department
    of Agriculture. 2015-2020 Dietary Guidelines for Americans. 8th
    Edition. December 2015. Cited 2017-01-05. Available from: URL:
    http://health.gov/dietaryguidelines/2015/ guidelines/

80  Elsenbruch S, Langhorst J, Popkirowa K, Müller T, Luedtke R,
    Franken U, Paul A, Spahn G, Michalsen A, Janssen OE, Schedlowski

M, Dobos GJ. Effects of mind-body therapy on quality of life and neuroendocrine and cellular immune functions in patients with ulcerative colitis. Psychother Psychosom 2005; 74: 277–287 [PMID: 16088265 DOI: 10.1159/000086318]

81    Dam AN, Berg AM, Farraye FA. Environmental influences on the onset and clinical course of Crohn's disease-part 1: an overview of external risk factors. Gastroenterol Hepatol (NY) 2013; 9: 711–717 [PMID: 24764788]

82    van Langenberg DR, Gibson PR. Factors associated with physical and cognitive fatigue in patients with Crohn's disease: a cross-sectional and longitudinal study. Inflamm Bowel Dis 2014; 20: 115–125 [PMID: 24297056 DOI: 10.1097/01. MIB.0000437614.91258.70]

83    van Langenberg DR, Gibson PR. Factors associated with physical and cognitive fatigue in patients with Crohn's disease: a cross-sectional and longitudinal study. Inflamm Bowel Dis 2014; 20: 115–125 [PMID: 24297056 DOI: 10.1097/01. MIB.0000437614.91258.70]

84    Bach-Faig A, Berry EM, Lairon D, Reguant J, Trichopoulou A, Dernini S, Medina FX, Battino M, Belahsen R, Miranda G, Serra-Majem L; Mediterranean Diet Foundation Expert Group. Mediterranean diet pyramid today. Science and cultural updates. Public Health Nutr 2011; 14: 2274–2284 [PMID: 22166184 DOI: 10.1017/S1368980011002515]

85    Gil A, Ruiz-Lopez MD, Fernandez-Gonzalez M, Martinez de Victoria E. The FINUT healthy lifestyles guide: Beyond the food pyramid. Adv Nutr 2014; 5: 358S–367S [PMID: 24829489 DOI: 10.3945/an.113.005637]

86    Grundmann O, Yoon SL. Complementary and alternative medicines in irritable bowel syndrome: an integrative view. World J Gastroenterol 2014; 20: 346–362 [PMID: 24574705 DOI: 10.3748/wjg.v20.i2.346]

87    Daley AJ, Grimmett C, Roberts L, Wilson S, Fatek M, Roalfe A, Singh S. The effects of exercise upon symptoms and quality of life in patients diagnosed with irritable bowel syndrome: a randomised controlled trial. Int J Sports Med 2008; 29: 778–782 [PMID: 18461499 DOI: 10.1055/s-2008-1038600]

88    Johannesson E, Ringström G, Abrahamsson H, Sadik R. Intervention to increase physical activity in irritable bowel syndrome shows

long-term positive effects. World J Gastroenterol 2015; 21: 600–608 [PMID: 25593485 DOI: 10.3748/wjg.v21. i2.600]

89 Kuttner L, Chambers CT, Hardial J, Israel DM, Jacobson K, Evans K. A randomized trial of yoga for adolescents with irritable bowel syndrome. Pain Res Manag 2006; 11: 217–223 [PMID: 17149454]

90 van Tilburg MA, Palsson OS, Levy RL, Feld AD, Turner MJ, Drossman DA, Whitehead WE. Complementary and alternative medicine use and cost in functional bowel disorders: a six month prospective study in a large HMO. BMC Complement Altern Med 2008; 8: 46 [PMID: 18652682 DOI: 10.1186/1472-6882-8-46]

91 Peters HP, De Vries WR, Vanberge-Henegouwen GP, Akkermans LM. Potential benefits and hazards of physical activity and exercise on the gastrointestinal tract. Gut 2001; 48: 435–439 [PMID:11171839]

92 Oettlé GJ. Effect of moderate exercise on bowel habit. Gut 1991; 32: 941–944 [PMID: 1885077]

93 de Oliveira EP, Burini RC. The impact of physical exercise on the gastrointestinal tract. Curr Opin Clin Nutr Metab Care 2009; 12: 533–538 [PMID: 19535976 DOI: 10.1097/ MCO.0b013e32832e6776]

94 Böhn L, Störsrud S, Törnblom H, Bengtsson U, Simrén M. Self-reported food-related gastrointestinal symptoms in IBS are common and associated with more severe symptoms and reduced quality of life. Am J Gastroenterol. 2013;108(5):634–641.

95 Lomer MC, Parkes GC, Sanderson JD. Review article: lactose intolerance in clinical practice – myths and realities. Aliment Pharmacol Ther. 2008;27(2):93–103.

96 Parker TJ, Woolner JT, Prevost AT, Tuffnell Q, Shorthouse M, Hunter JO. Irritable bowel syndrome: is the search for lactose intolerance justified? Eur J Gastroenterol Hepatol. 2001;13(3):219–225.

97 Böhmer CJ, Tuynman HA. The clinical relevance of lactose malabsorption in irritable bowel syndrome. Eur J Gastroenterol Hepatol. 1996;8(10):1013–1016.

98 Hoveyda N, Heneghan C, Mahtani KR, Perera R, Roberts N, Glasziou P. A systematic review and meta-analysis: probiotics in the treatment of irritable bowel syndrome. BMC Gastroenterol. 2009;9:15.

99 Lenhart A, Ferch C, Shaw M, Chey W.D. Use of dietary management in irritable Bowel Syndrome: results of a survey

of over 1500 United States Gastroenterologists. Journal of Neurogastroenterology and Motility. 2018; 24 (3):437–446. https://doi.org/10.5056/jnm17116.

100   Central Clinical School, Monash University and The Alfred Hospital. The Monash University Low FODMAP Diet. 4th ed. Melbourne, Australia: Monash University; 2012.

101   Barrett JS, Gibson PR. Clinical ramifications of malabsorption of fructose and other short-chain carbohydrates. Pract Gastroenterol. 2007; 31:51–65.

102   Notes: Data from Monash University. Low FODMAP Diet Application. Available at: http://www.med.monash.edu/cecs/gastro/fodmap/. Android version accessed August 26, 2015.72 Abbreviations: FODMAP, fermentable oligosaccharide, disaccharide, monosaccharide, and polyols; FOS, fructo-oligosaccharides; GOS, galacto-oligosaccharides.)

103   Shepherd SJ, Lomer MC, Gibson PR. Short-chain carbohydrates and functional gastrointestinal disorders. Am J Gastroenterol. 2013; 108:707–17. This review provides comprehensive evaluation of FODMAPs in functional gastrointestinal disorders. [PubMed: 23588241]

104   Kim Y, Park SC, Wolf BW, Hertzler SR. Combination of erythritol and fructose increases gastrointestinal symptoms in healthy adults. Nutr Res. 2011; 31:836–41.

105   Fernández-Bañares F, Esteve M, Viver JM. Fructose-sorbitol malabsorption. Curr Gastroenterol Rep. 2009; 11:368–74.

106   Fedewa E, Rao S.S.C. Dietary fructose intolerance, fructan intolerance and FODMAPs. Curr Gastroenterol Rep. 2014; 16(1): 370. doi:10.1007/s11894-013-0370-0.

107   Tuck CJ, Muir JG, Barrett JS, Gibson PR. Fermentable oligosaccharides, disaccharides, monosaccharides and polyols: role in irritable bowel syndrome. Expert Rev Gastroenterol Hepatol. 2014;8(7):819–834.

108   Murray K, Wilkinson-Smith V, Hoad C, et al. Differential effects of FODMAPs (fermentable oligo-, di-, mono-saccharides and polyols) on small and large intestinal contents in healthy subjects shown by MRI. Am J Gastroenterol. 2014;109(1):110–119.

109   Halmos EP, Power VA, Shepherd SJ, Gibson PR, Muir JG. A diet
      low in FODMAPs reduces symptoms of irritable bowel syndrome.
      Gastroenterology. 2014;146(1):67–75.e5.

110   Vanhoutvin SA, Troost FJ, Kilkens TO, et al. The effects of
      butyrate enemas on visceral perception in healthy volunteers.
      Neurogastroenterol Motil. 2009;21(9):952–957, e76.

111   McIntosh K, Reed DE, Schneider T, et al. FODMAPs alter
      symptoms and the metabolome of patients with IBS: a randomised
      controlled trial [published online March 14, 2016]. Gut.
      doi:10.1136/gutjnl-2015-311339.

112   Camilleri, M.; Boeckxstaens, G. Dietary and pharmacological
      treatment of abdominal pain in IBS. Gut 2017, 66, 966–974.
      [CrossRef] [PubMed]

113   Böhn, L.; Störsrud, S.; Liljebo, T.; Collin, L.; Lindfors, P.; Törnblom,
      H.; Simrén, M. Diet low in FODMAPs reduces symptoms of
      irritable bowel syndrome as well as traditional dietary advice: A
      randomized controlled trial. Gastroenterology 2015, 149, 1399–
      1407. [CrossRef] [PubMed]

114   Gibson, P.R. The evidence base for efficacy of the low FODMAP
      diet in irritable bowel syndrome: Is it ready for prime time as a first-
      line therapy? J. Gastroenterol. Hepatol. 2017, 32, 32–35. [CrossRef]
      [PubMed]

115   Gibson, P.R.; Shepherd, S.J. Evidence-based dietary management of
      functional gastrointestinal symptoms: The FODMAP approach. J.
      Gastroenterol. Hepatol. 2010, 25, 252–258. [CrossRef] [PubMed]

116   Valeur, J.; Røseth, A.G.; Knudsen, T.; Malmstrøm, G.H.; Fiennes,
      J.T.; Midtvedt, T.; Berstad, A. Fecal Fermentation in Irritable
      Bowel Syndrome: Influence of Dietary Restriction of Fermentable
      Oligosaccharides, Disaccharides, Monosaccharides and Polyols.
      Digestion 2016, 94, 50–56. [CrossRef] [PubMed]

117   Hustoft, T.N.; Hausken, T.; Ystad, S.O.; Valeur, J.; Brokstad, K.;
      Hatlebakk, J.G.; Lied, G.A. Effects of varying dietary content
      of fermentable short-chain carbohydrates on symptoms, fecal
      microenvironment, and cytokine profiles in patients with irritable
      bowel syndrome. Neurogastroenterol. Motil. 2017. [CrossRef]
      [PubMed]

118   Staudacher, H.M.; Whelan, K. Altered gastrointestinal microbiota
      in irritable bowel syndrome and its modification by diet: Probiotics,
      prebiotics and the low FODMAP diet. Proc. Nutr. Soc. 2016, 75,
      306–318. [CrossRef] [PubMed]

119   Shepherd, S.J.; Lomer, M.C.; Gibson, P.R. Short-chain carbohydrates
      and functional gastrointestinal disorders. Am. J. Gastroenterol.
      2013, 108, 707–717. [CrossRef] [PubMed]

120   Chumpitazi, B.P.; Cope, J.L.; Hollister, E.B.; Tsai, C.M.; McMeans,
      A.R.; Luna, R.A.; Versalovic, J.; Shulman, R.J. Randomised clinical
      trial: Gut microbiome biomarkers are associated with clinical
      response to a low FODMAP diet in children with the irritable
      bowel syndrome. Aliment. Pharmacol. Ther. 2015, 42, 418–427.
      [CrossRef] [PubMed]

121   Nanayakkara WS, Skidmore PM, O'Brien L, Wilkinson TJ,
      Gearry RB. Efficacy of the low FODMAP diet for treating irritable
      bowel syndrome: the evidence to date. Clin Exp Gastroenterol.
      2016;9:131–142.

122   Kinrade SK, Twamley RM, Fell L, et al. An audit to assess feasiblity
      and efficacy of group education for irritable bowel syndrome
      (IBS) patients in the delivery of low FODMAP (fermentatble
      oligosaccharides, disaccharides, monosaccharides and polyols)
      dietary advice. Gut. 2014;63(suppl 1):A238.

123   Monash University. Low FODMAP diet for irritable bowel
      syndrome. Available at http://www.med.monash.edu/cecs/gastro/
      fodmap/. Accessed September 20, 2016.

124   Hill P, Muir J.G, Ginson P.R. Controversies and recent developments
      of the low-FODMAP diet. Gastroenterology & Hepatology. 2017;
      13 (1):36–45.

125   Staudacher HM, Whelan K, Irving PM, Lomer MC. Comparison
      of symptom response following advice for a diet low in fermentable
      carbohydrates (FODMAPs) versus standard dietary advice
      in patients with irritable bowel syndrome. J Hum Nutr Diet.
      2011;24(5):487–495.

126   Marsh A, Eslick EM, Eslick GD. Does a diet low in FODMAPs
      reduce symptoms associated with functional gastrointestinal
      disorders? A comprehensive systematic review and meta-analysis.
      Eur J Nutr. 2016;55(3):897–906.

127 Eswaran SL, Chey WD, Han-Markey T, Ball S, Jackson K. A randomized controlled trial comparing the low FODMAP diet vs. modified NICE guidelines in US adults with IBS-D. Am J Gastroenterol. 2016;111(12):1824–1832.

128 Peters SL, Yao CK, Philpott H, Yelland GW, Muir JG, Gibson PR. Randomised clinical trial: the efficacy of gut-directed hypnotherapy is similar to that of the low FODMAP diet for the treatment of irritable bowel syndrome. Aliment Pharmacol Ther. 2016;44(5):447–459.

129 Laatikainen R, Koskenpato J, Hongisto SM, et al. Randomised clinical trial: low-FODMAP rye bread vs. regular rye bread to relieve the symptoms of irritable bowel syndrome. Aliment Pharmacol Ther. 2016;44(5):460–470.

130 Peters SL, Muir JG, Gibson PR. Review article: gut-directed hypnotherapy in the management of irritable bowel syndrome and inflammatory bowel disease. Aliment Pharmacol Ther. 2015;41(11):1104–1115.

131 De Giorgio R, Volta U, Gibson PR. Sensitivity to wheat, gluten and FODMAPs in IBS: facts or fiction? Gut. 2016;65(1):169–178.

132 Golley S, Corsini N, Topping D, Morell M, Mohr P. Motivations for avoiding wheat consumption in Australia: results from a population survey. Public Health Nutr. 2015;18(3):490–499.

133 Gibson PR, Muir JG. Not all effects of a gluten-free diet are due to removal of gluten. Gastroenterology. 2013;145(3):693.

134 Aziz I, Trott N, Briggs R, North JR, Hadjivassiliou M, Sanders DS. Efficacy of a gluten-free diet in subjects with irritable bowel syndrome-diarrhea unaware of their HLA-DQ2/8 genotype. Clin Gastroenterol Hepatol. 2016;14(5):696–703.e1.

135 Austin GL, Dalton CB, Hu Y, et al. A very low-carbohydrate diet improves symptoms and quality of life in diarrhea-predominant irritable bowel syndrome. Clin Gastroenterol Hepatol. 2009;7(6):706–708.e1.

136 Vazquez-Roque MI, Camilleri M, Smyrk T, et al. A controlled trial of glutenfree diet in patients with irritable bowel syndrome-diarrhea: effects on bowel frequency and intestinal function. Gastroenterology. 2013;144(5):903–911.e3.

137   Molina-Infante J, Santolaria S, Sanders DS, Fernández-Bañares F. Systematic review: noncoeliac gluten sensitivity. Aliment Pharmacol Ther. 2015;41(9):807–820.

138   Biesiekierski JR, Newnham ED, Shepherd SJ, Muir JG, Gibson PR. Characterization of adults with a self-diagnosis of non-celiac gluten sensitivity. Nutr Clin Pract. 2014;29(4):504–509.

139   Biesiekierski JR, Peters SL, Newnham ED, Rosella O, Muir JG, Gibson PR. No effects of gluten in patients with self-reported non-celiac gluten sensitivity after dietary reduction of fermentable, poorly absorbed, short-chain carbohydrates. Gastroenterology. 2013;145(2):320–328.e1–3.

140   Di Sabatino A, Volta U, Salvatore C, et al. Small amounts of gluten in subjects with suspected nonceliac gluten sensitivity: a randomized, double-blind, placebocontrolled, cross-over trial. Clin Gastroenterol Hepatol. 2015;13(9):1604–12.e3.

141   Elli L, Tomba C, Branchi F, et al. Evidence for the presence of non-celiac gluten sensitivity in patients with functional gastrointestinal symptoms: results from a multicenter randomized double-blind placebo-controlled gluten challenge. Nutrients. 2016;8(2):84.

142   Lomer MCE. Review article: the aetiology, diagnosis, mechanisms and clinical evidence for food intolerance. Aliment Pharmacol Ther. 2015;41(3):262–275. 36. Rao SS, Attaluri A, Anderson L, Stumbo P. Ability of the normal human small intestine to absorb fructose: evaluation by breath testing. Clin Gastroenterol Hepatol. 2007;5(8):959–963.

143   Rao SS, Attaluri A, Anderson L, Stumbo P. Ability of the normal human small intestine to absorb fructose: evaluation by breath testing. Clin Gastroenterol Hepatol. 2007;5(8):959–963.

144   Yao CK, Tuck CJ, Barrett JS, et al. Poor reproducibility of breath hydrogen testing: implications for its application in functional bowel disorders. United European Gastroenterol J. In press.

145   Yao CK, Tan HL, van Langenberg DR, et al. Dietary sorbitol and mannitol: food content and distinct absorption patterns between healthy individuals and patients with irritable bowel syndrome. J Hum Nutr Diet. 2014;27(suppl 2):263–275.

146   Saps M, Nichols-Vinueza DX, Rosen JM, Velasco-Benítez CA. Prevalence of functional gastrointestinal disorders in Colombian school children. J Pediatr. 2014;164(3):542–545.e1.

147   Devanarayana NM, Adhikari C, Pannala W, Rajindrajith S. Prevalence of functional gastrointestinal diseases in a cohort of Sri Lankan adolescents: comparison between Rome II and Rome III criteria. J Trop Pediatr. 2011;57(1):34–39.

148   Youssef NN, Murphy TG, Langseder AL, Rosh JR. Quality of life for children with functional abdominal pain: a comparison study of patients' and parents' perceptions. Pediatrics. 2006;117(1):54–59.

149   Youssef NN, Atienza K, Langseder AL, Strauss RS. Chronic abdominal pain and depressive symptoms: analysis of the national longitudinal study of adolescent health. Clin Gastroenterol Hepatol. 2008;6(3):329–332.

150   Dhroove G, Chogle A, Saps M. A million-dollar work-up for abdominal pain: is it worth it? J Pediatr Gastroenterol Nutr. 2010;51(5):579–583.

151   Horst S, Shelby G, Anderson J, et al. Predicting persistence of functional abdominal pain from childhood into young adulthood. Clin Gastroenterol Hepatol. 2014;12(12):2026–2032.

152   Hyams JS, Leichtner AM. Apple juice. An unappreciated cause of chronic diarrhea. Am J Dis Child. 1985;139(5):503–505.

153   Gomara RE, Halata MS, Newman LJ, et al. Fructose intolerance in children presenting with abdominal pain. J Pediatr Gastroenterol Nutr. 2008;47(3): 303–308.

154   Escobar MAJ Jr, Lustig D, Pflugeisen BM, et al. Fructose intolerance/malabsorption and recurrent abdominal pain in children. J Pediatr Gastroenterol Nutr. 2014;58(4):498–501.

155   Wintermeyer P, Baur M, Pilic D, Schmidt-Choudhury A, Zilbauer M, Wirth S. Fructose malabsorption in children with recurrent abdominal pain: positive effects of dietary treatment. Klin Padiatr. 2012;224(1):17–21.

156   Däbritz J, Mühlbauer M, Domagk D, et al. Significance of hydrogen breath tests in children with suspected carbohydrate malabsorption. BMC Pediatr. 2014;14:59.

157  Jones HF, Burt E, Dowling K, Davidson G, Brooks DA, Butler
     RN. Effect of age on fructose malabsorption in children presenting
     with gastrointestinal symptoms. J Pediatr Gastroenterol Nutr.
     2011;52(5):581–584.

158  Wirth S, Klodt C, Wintermeyer P, et al. Positive or negative fructose
     breath test results do not predict response to fructose restricted diet
     in children with recurrent abdominal pain: results from a prospective
     randomized trial. Klin Padiatr. 2014;226(5):268–273.

159  Bratten JR, Spanier J, Jones MP. Lactulose breath testing does not
     discriminate patients with irritable bowel syndrome from healthy
     controls. Am J Gastroenterol. 2008;103(4):958–963.

160  Chogle A, Mintjens S, Saps M. Pediatric IBS: an overview
     on pathophysiology, diagnosis and treatment. Pediatr Ann.
     2014;43(4):e76-e82.

161  https://www.monashfodmap.com/ibs-central/i-have-ibs/
     starting-the-low-fodmap-diet/

162  Gibson PR. How to treat: irritable bowel syndrome. Australian
     Doctor. 2012;133:27–41.

163  Staudacher HM, Lomer MC, Anderson JL, et al. Fermentable
     carbohydrate restriction reduces luminal bifidobacteria and
     gastrointestinal symptoms in patients with irritable bowel syndrome.
     J Nutr. 2012;142(8):1510–1518.

164  Halmos EP, Christophersen CT, Bird AR, Shepherd SJ, Gibson
     PR, Muir JG. Diets that differ in their FODMAP content alter the
     colonic luminal microenvironment. Gut. 2015;64(1):93–100.

165  Kerckhoffs AP, Samsom M, van der Rest ME, et al. Lower
     Bifidobacteria counts in both duodenal mucosa-associated and
     fecal microbiota in irritable bowel syndrome patients. World J
     Gastroenterol. 2009;15(23):2887–2892.

166  Parkes GC, Rayment NB, Hudpith BN, et al. Distinct microbial
     populations exist in the mucosa-associated microbiota of sub-
     groups of irritable bowel syndrome. Neurogastroenterol Motil.
     2012;24(1):31–39.

167  Mättö J, Maunuksela L, Kajander, K et al. Composition and
     temporal stability of gastrointestinal microbiota in irritable bowel
     syndrome—a longitudinal study in IBS and control subjects. FEMS
     Immunol Med Microbiol. 2005;43(2):213–222.

168  Manichanh C, Eck A, Varela E, et al. Anal gas evacuation and colonic microbiota in patients with flatulence: effect of diet. Gut. 2014;63(3):401–408.

169  Satherley R, Howard R, Higgs S. Disordered eating practices in gastrointestinal disorders. Appetite. 2015;84:240–250.

170  Dunn TM, Bratman S. On orthorexia nervosa: a review of the literature and proposed diagnostic criteria. Eat Behav. 2016;21:11–17.

171  Aleksandrova K, Mosquera B. R, Hernandez V. Diet, Gut Microbiome and epigenetics: emerging links with inflammatory bowel diseases and prospects for management and prevention. Nutrients. 2017;9: 962. doi:10.3390/nu9090962.

172  http://www.med.monash.edu/cecs/gastro/fodmap/. Android version accessed August 26, 2015.72

173  Nanayakkara W.S, Skidmore P. ML, Brien L.O, Wilkinson T.H, Gearry R.B. Efficacy of the low FODMAP diet for treating irritable bowel syndrome: the evidence to date. Clinical and Experimental Gastroenterology. 2016; 9:131–142. http://dx.doi.org/10.2147/CEG.S86798.

174  Longstreth GF, Thompson WG, Chey WD, Houghton LA, Mearin F, Spiller RC. Functional bowel disorders. Gastroenterology. 2006;130(5):1480–1491.

175  Wong RK, Palsson OS, Turner MJ, et al. Inability of the Rome III criteria to distinguish functional constipation from constipation-subtype irritable bowel syndrome. Am J Gastroenterol. 2010;105(10):2228–2234.

176  Heidelbaugh JJ, Stelwagon M, Miller SA, Shea EP, Chey WD. The spectrum of constipation-predominant irritable bowel syndrome and chronic idiopathic constipation: US survey assessing symptoms, care seeking, and disease burden. Am J Gastroenterol. 2015;110(4):580–587.

177  Bharucha AE, Locke GR, Zinsmeister AR, et al. Differences between painless and painful constipation among community women. Am J Gastroenterol. 2006;101(3):604–612.

178  Drossman DA, Morris C, Hu Y, et al. Further characterization of painful constipation (PC): clinical features over one year and comparison with IBS. J Clin Gastroenterol. 2008;42(10):1080–1088.

179  Rey E, Balboa A, Mearin F. Chronic constipation, irritable
     bowel syndrome with constipation and constipation with pain/
     discomfort: similarities and differences. Am J Gastroenterol.
     2014;109(6):876–884.

180  Shekhar C, Monaghan PJ, Morris J, et al. Rome III functional
     constipation and irritable bowel syndrome with constipation are
     similar disorders within a spectrum of sensitization, regulated by
     serotonin. Gastroenterology. 2013;145(4):749–757; quiz e13-e14.

181  Zhao YF, Ma XQ, Wang R, et al. Epidemiology of functional
     constipation and comparison with constipation-predominant
     irritable bowel syndrome: the Systematic Investigation of
     Gastrointestinal Diseases in China (SILC). Aliment Pharmacol Ther.
     2011;34(8):1020–1029.

182  Koloski NA, Jones M, Young M, Talley NJ. Differentiation of
     functional constipation and constipation predominant irritable
     bowel syndrome based on Rome III criteria: a population-based
     study. Aliment Pharmacol Ther. 2015;41(9):856–866.

183  Nellesen D, Chawla A, Oh DL, Weissman T, Lavins BJ, Murray
     CW. Comorbidities in patients with irritable bowel syndrome with
     constipation or chronic idiopathic constipation: a review of the
     literature from the past decade. Postgrad Med. 2013;125(2):40–50.

184  Lacy BE, Mearin F, Chang L, et al. Bowel disorders.
     Gastroenterology 2016;150:1393–407.

185  Bharucha AE, Pemberton JH, Locke GR 3rd. American
     Gastroenterological Association technical review on constipation.
     Gastroenterology 2013;144:218–238

186  Grundy D, Al-Chaer ED, Aziz Q, et al. Fundamentals of
     neurogastroenterology: basic science. Gastroenterology 2006;
     130:1391–1411.

187  Rao SS. Constipation: evaluation and treatment of colonic and
     anorectal motility disorders. Gastrointest Endosc Clin N Am
     2009;19:117–139, vii. 8. Drossman DA. Functional gastrointestinal
     disorders: History, pathophysiology, clinical features and Rome IV.
     Gastroenterology 2016.

188  Lembo A, Camilleri M. Chronic constipation. N Engl J Med
     2003;349:1360–1368.

189  Pyleris E, Giamarellos-Bourboulis EJ, Tzivras D, Koussoulas V, Barbatzas C, Pimentel M. The prevalence of overgrowth by aerobic bacteria in the small intestine by small bowel culture: relationship with irritable bowel syndrome. Dig Dis Sci 2012;57:1321–1329

190  American Gastroenterological A, Bharucha AE, Dorn SD, Lembo A, Pressman A. American Gastroenterological Association medical position statement on constipation. Gastroenterology 2013;144:211–217.

191  Drossman DA. Functional gastrointestinal disorders: History, pathophysiology, clinical features and Rome IV. Gastroenterology 2016.

192  Gallegos-Orozco JF, Foxx-Orenstein AE, Sterler SM, Stoa JM. Chronic constipation in the elderly. Am J Gastroenterol 2012; 107:18–26.

193  Mancini I, Bruera E. Constipation in advanced cancer patients. Support Care Cancer 1998; 6:356–364.

194  Bassotti G, Chistolini F, Sietchiping-Nzepa F, de Roberto G, Morelli A, Chiarioni G. Biofeedback for pelvic floor dysfunction in constipation. BMJ 2004; 328:393–396.

195  Mearin F, Ciriza C, Mínguez M, Rey E, Mascort J.J, Peña E, Cañones P, Júdez J. Clinical Practice Guideline: Irritable bowel syndrome with constipation and functional constipation in the adult. Rev Esp Enferm Dig (Madrid). 2016; 108 (6):332–363.

196  Krogh K, Chiarioni G, Whitehead W. Management of chronic constipation in adults. United European Gastroenterology Journal. 2017; 5(4): 465–472.

197  Jani B, Marsicano E. Constipation: Evaluati on and Management. Missouri Medicine. 2018;115 (3): 236–240.

198  Bharucha AE, Dorn SD, Lembo A, Pressman A; American Gastroenterological Association. American Gastroenterological Association medical position statement on constipation. Gastroenterology. 2013;144(1):211–217.

199  Chiarioni G, Kim SM, Vantini I, Whitehead WE. Validation of the balloon evacuation test: reproducibility and agreement with findings from anorectal manometry and electromyography. Clin Gastroenterol Hepatol. 2014;12(12):2049–2054.

200 Lembo A, Camilleri M. Chronic constipation. N Engl J Med. 2003;349(14): 1360–1368.

201 Nyam DC, Pemberton JH, Ilstrup DM, Rath DM. Long-term results of surgery for chronic constipation. Dis Colon Rectum. 1997;40(3):273–279.

202 Chiarioni G, Kim SM, Whitehead WE. Overlap of IBS with normal transit constipation but not dyssynergic defecation. Gastroenterology. 2013;144(5 suppl 1): S-726.

203 Bouin M, Plourde V, Boivin M, et al. Rectal distention testing in patients with irritable bowel syndrome: sensitivity, specificity, and predictive values of pain sensory thresholds. Gastroenterology. 2002;122(7):1771–1777.

204 Suttor VP, Prott GM, Hansen RD, Kellow JE, Malcolm A. Evidence for pelvic floor dyssynergia in patients with irritable bowel syndrome. Dis Colon Rectum. 2010;53(2):156–160.

205 American Gastroenterological Association, Bharucha AE, Dorn SD, Lembo A, Pressman A. American Gastroenterological Association medical position statement on constipation. Gastroenterology 2013; 144:211–217.

206 Costilla VC, Foxx-Orenstein AE. Constipation in adults: diagnosis and management. Curr Treat Options Gastroenterol 2014; 12:310–321.

207 El-Serag HB, Olden K, Bjorkman D. Health-related quality of life among persons with irritable bowel syndrome: A systematic review. Alimentary Pharmacology & Therapeutics 2002;16(6):1171–85. PMID: 12030961. DOI: 10.1046/j.1365-2036.2002.01290.x

208 Mearin F, Perello A, Perona M. Quality of life in patients with irritable bowel syndrome. Gastroenterología y Hepatología 2004;27(Suppl.3):24–31. DOI: 10.1157/13058927

209 Everhart JE, Ruhl CE. Burden of digestive diseases in the United States Part II: Lower gastrointestinal diseases. Gastroenterology 2009;136(3):741–54. PMID: 19166855. DOI: 10.1053/j. gastro.2009.01.015

210 Johanson JF, Kralstein J. Chronic constipation: A survey of the patient perspective. Alimentary Pharmacology & Therapeutics 2007;25(5):599–608. PMID: 17305761. DOI: 10.1111/j.13652036. 2006.03238.x

211  Sanchez MI, Bercik P. Epidemiology and burden of chronic
     constipation. Can J Gastroenterol 2011;25: 11B-L 15B.

212  Mounsey A, Raleigh M, Wilson A. Management of constipation in
     older adults. American Family Physician. 2015; 92 (6): 500–504.

213  Tack J, Müller-Lissner S, Stanghellini V. Diagnosis and treatment of
     chronic constipation–a European perspective. Neurogastroenterol
     Motil. 2011;23:697–710

214  Menees SB, Guentner A, Chey SW, Saad R, Chey WD. How Do
     US Gastroenterologists Use Over-the-Counter and Prescription
     Medications in Patients With Gastroesophageal Reflux and Chronic
     Constipation?. Am J Gastroenterol 2015, in press.

215  Harari D. Constipation. In: Halter JB, Ouslander JG, Tinetti ME,
     editors. Hazzard's Geriatric Medicine and Gerontology. 6th ed. New
     York, USA: McGraw-Hill Companies; 2009. p. 1103–22.

216  Andersson H, Bosaeus I, Falkheden T, Melkersson M. Transit
     time in constipated geriatric patients during treatment with a
     bulk laxative and bran: a comparison. Scand J Gastroenterol.
     1979;14:821–6.

217  Nour-Eldein H, Salama HM, Abdulmajeed AA, Heissam KS. The
     effect of lifestyle modification on severity of constipation and quality
     of life of elders in nursing homes at Ismailia city, Egypt. J Family
     Community Med. 2014;21:100–6.

218  Ford AC, Moayyedi P, Lacy BE, et al. American College of
     Gastroenterology Monograph on the Management of Irritable
     Bowel Syndrome and Chronic Idiopathic Constipation. Am J
     Gastroenterol. 2014;109:S2–26.

219  Spinzi G, Amato A, Imperiali G, et al. Constipation in the elderly:
     management strategies. Drugs Aging. 2009;26:469–74.

220  Miller LE, Ouwehand AC. Probiotic supplementation decreases
     intestinal transit time: meta-analysis of randomized controlled trials.
     World J Gastroenterol. 2013;19:4718–25.

221  Dietz HP. Rectocele or stool quality: what matters more for
     symptoms of obstructed defecation? Tech Coloproctol 2009; 13:
     265–268 [PMID: 19685268 DOI: 10.1007/s10151-009-0527-x]

222  Drummond L, Gearry RB. Kiwifruit modulation of gastrointestinal
     motility. Adv Food Nutr Res 2013;68:219–32.

223 Na JR, Oh KN, Park SU, Bae D, Choi EJ, Jung MA, et al. The laxative effects of Maesil (Prunus mume Siebold & Zucc.) on constipation induced by a low-fibre diet in a rat model. Int J Food Sci Nutr 2013;64:333–45.

224 Bubba MD, Giordani E, Pippucci L, Cincinelli A, Checchini L, Galvan P. Changes in tannins, ascorbic acid and sugar content in astringent persimmons during on-tree growth and ripening and in response to different postharvest treatments. J Food Compos Anal 2009;22:668–77.

225 Bassotti G, Chiarioni G, Vantini I, et al. Anorectal manometric abnormalities and colonic propulsive impairment in patients with severe chronic idiopathic constipation. Dig Dis Sci. 1994;39:1558–64.

226 Ford AC, Talley NJ, Spiegel BM, et al. Effect of fibre, antispasmodics, and peppermint oil in the treatment of irritable bowel syndrome: systematic review and meta-analysis. BMJ 2008; 337:a2313.

227 Wall GC, Bryant GA, Bottenberg MM, Maki ED, Miesner AR. Irritable bowel syndrome: a concise review of current treatment concepts. World J Gastroenterol 2014; 20:8796–8806

228 Kligler B, Chaudhary S. Peppermint oil. Am Fam Physician 2007; 75:1027–1030.

229 Bassotti G, Chiarioni G, Vantini I, et al. Anorectal manometric abnormalities and colonic propulsive impairment in patients with severe chronic idiopathic constipation. Dig Dis Sci. 1994;39:1558–64

230 van den Berg MM, Benninga MA, Di Lorenzo C. Epidemiology of childhood constipation: A systematic review. Am J Gastroenterol 2006;101(10):2401–09.

231 Paul SP, Broad SR, Spray C. Idiopathic constipation in children clinical practice guidelines. Arch Dis Child Educ Pract Ed 2016;101(2):65–69.

232 Mugie SM, Benninga MA, Di Lorenzo C. Epidemiology of constipation in children and adults: a systematic review. Best Pract Res Clin Gastroenterol 2011; 25: 3–18 [PMID: 21382575 DOI: 10.1016/j.bpg.2010.12.010]

233 Lu PL, Saps M, Chanis RA, Velasco-Benitez CA. The prevalence of functional gastrointestinal disorders in children in Panama: a schoolbased study. Acta Paediatr. 2016;105(5):e232–e236.

234  Zhang SC, Wang WL, Qu RB, et al. Epidemiologic survey on the prevalence and distribution of childhood functional constipation in the northern areas of China: a population-based study. Zhonghua Liu Xing Bing Xue Za Zhi. 2010;31(7):751–754. Chinese.

235  Bhatia V, Deswal S, Seth S, Kapoor A, Sibal A, Gopalan S. Prevalence of functional gastrointestinal disorders among adolescents in Delhi based on Rome III criteria: a school-based survey. Indian J Gastroenterol. 2016;35(4):294–298.

236  Lewis ML, Palsson OS, Whitehead WE, van Tilburg MA. Prevalence of functional gastrointestinal disorders in children and adolescents. J Pediatr. 2016;177:39–43.e3.

237  Vandenplas Y, Abkari A, Bellaiche M, et al. Prevalence and health outcomes of functional gastrointestinal symptoms in infants from birth to 12 months of age. J Pediatr Gastroenterol Nutr. 2015;61(5):531–537.

238  van Tilburg MA, Hyman PE, Walker L, et al. Prevalence of functional gastrointestinal disorders in infants and toddlers. J Pediatr. 2015;166(3):684–689.

239  Boccia G, Manguso F, Coccorullo P, Masi P, Pensabene L, Staiano A. Functional defecation disorders in children: PACCT criteria versus Rome II criteria. J Pediatr. 2007;151(4):394–398, 398 e1.

240  Lu PL, Saps M, Chanis RA, Velasco-Benitez CA. The prevalence of functional gastrointestinal disorders in children in Panama: a schoolbased study. Acta Paediatr. 2016;105(5):e232–e236.

241  Walter HA, Hovenkamp A, Rajindrajith S, Devanarayana NM, Rajapakshe NN, Benninga MA. OP-12 prevalence of functional constipation in infants and toddlers in Sri Lanka. J Pediatr Gastroenterol Nutr. 2015;61(4):541.

242  Rajindrajith S, Devanarayana NM. Constipation in children: novel insight into epidemiology, pathophysiology and management. J Neurogastroenterol Motil. 2011;17(1):35–47.

243  Knowles CH, Farrugia G. Gastrointestinal neuromuscular pathology in chronic constipation. Best Pract Res Clin Gastroenterol. 2011;25(1): 43–57.

244  Mehta M, Beg M. Fructose intolerance: cause or cure of chronic functional constipation. Global Pediatric Health. 2018; 5: 1–5. https://doi.org/10.1177/2333794X18761460.

245   Lewis SJ, Heaton KW. Stool form scale as a useful guide to intestinal transit time. Scand J Gastroenterol. 1997;32(9):920–924.

246   Waterham M, Kaufman J, Gibb S. Childhood constipation. Australian Family Physician (AFP). 2017; 46 (12): 908–912.

247   Rajindrajith S, Devanarayana N.M, Perera B.J.C, Benninga M.A. Childhood constipation as an emerging public health problem. World Journal of Gastroenterolgy. 2016; 22(30): 6864–6875. DOI: 10.3748/wjg.v22.i30.6864.

248   Devanarayana NM, Rajindrajith S. Association between constipation and stressful life events in a cohort of Sri Lankan children and adolescents. J Trop Pediatr 2010; 56: 144–148 [PMID: 19696192 DOI: 10.1093/tropej/fmp077]

249   Inan M, Aydiner CY, Tokuc B, Aksu B, Ayvaz S, Ayhan S, Ceylan T, Basaran UN. Factors associated with childhood constipation. J Paediatr Child Health 2007; 43: 700–706 [PMID: 17640287]

250   Tam YH, Li AM, So HK, Shit KY, Pang KK, Wong YS, Tsui SY, Mou JW, Chan KW, Lee KH. Socioenvironmental factors associated with constipation in Hong Kong children and Rome III criteria. J Pediatr Gastroenterol Nutr 2012; 55: 56–61 [PMID: 22197949 DOI: 10.1097/MPG.0b013e31824741ce]

251   Rajindrajith S, Mettananda S, Devanarayana NM. Constipation during and after the civil war in Sri Lanka: a paediatric study. J Trop Pediatr 2011; 57: 439–443 [PMID: 21325393 DOI: 10.1093/ tropej/ fmr013]

252   Klooker TK, Braak B, Painter RC, de Rooij SR, van Elburg RM, van den Wijngaard RM, Roseboom TJ, Boeckxstaens GE. Exposure to severe wartime conditions in early life is associated with an increased risk of irritable bowel syndrome: a populationbased cohort study. Am J Gastroenterol 2009; 104: 2250–2256 [PMID: 19513027 DOI: 10.1038/ajg.2009.282]

253   Videlock EJ, Adeyemo M, Licudine A, Hirano M, Ohning G, Mayer M, Mayer EA, Chang L. Childhood trauma is associated with hypothalamic-pituitary-adrenal axis responsiveness in irritable bowel syndrome. Gastroenterology 2009; 137: 1954–1962 [PMID: 19737564 DOI: 10.1053/j.gastro.2009.08.058]

254   van Dijk M, de Vries GJ, Last BF, Benninga MA, Grootenhuis MA. Parental child-rearing attitudes are associated with functional

constipation in childhood. Arch Dis Child 2015; 100: 329–333
[PMID: 25359759 DOI: 10.1136/archdischild-2014-305941]

255  Gilbert R, Widom CS, Browne K, Fergusson D, Webb E, Janson
S. Burden and consequences of child maltreatment in high-income
countries. Lancet 2009; 373: 68–81 [PMID: 19056114 DOI:
10.1016/S0140-6736(08)61706-7]

256  Akmatov MK. Child abuse in 28 developing and transitional
countries--results from the Multiple Indicator Cluster Surveys. Int
J Epidemiol 2011; 40: 219–227 [PMID: 20943933 DOI: 10.1093/
ije/dyq168]

257  Rajindrajith S, Devanarayana NM, Lakmini C, Subasinghe V, de
Silva DG, Benninga MA. Association between child maltreatment
and constipation: a school-based survey using Rome III criteria. J
Pediatr Gastroenterol Nutr 2014; 58: 486–490 [PMID: 24253365
DOI: 10.1097/MPG.0000000000000249]

258  Chang L. The role of stress on physiologic responses and clinical
symptoms in irritable bowel syndrome. Gastroenterology
2011; 140: 761–765 [PMID: 21256129 DOI: 10.1053/j.
gastro.2011.01.032]

259  Dehghani SM, Moravej H, Rajaei E, Javaherizadeh H. Evaluation of
familial aggregation, vegetable consumption, legumes consumption,
and physical activity on functional constipation in families of
children with functional constipation versus children without
constipation. Prz Gastroenterol 2015; 10: 89–93 [PMID: 26557939
DOI: 10.5114/pg.2015.48996]

260  Ostwani W, Dolan J, Elitsur Y. Familial clustering of habitual
constipation: a prospective study in children from West Virginia. J
Pediatr Gastroenterol Nutr 2010; 50: 287–289 [PMID: 19668012
DOI: 10.1097/MPG.0b013e3181a0a595]

261  Peeters B, Benninga MA, Hennekam RC. Childhood constipation;
an overview of genetic studies and associated syndromes. Best Pract
Res Clin Gastroenterol 2011; 25: 73–88 [PMID: 21382580 DOI:
10.1016/j.bpg.2010.12.005]

262  Benninga MA, Voskuijl WP, Akkerhuis GW, Taminiau JA, Büller
HA. Colonic transit times and behaviour profiles in children with
defecation disorders. Arch Dis Child 2004; 89: 13–16 [PMID:
14709493]

263  Ranasinghe N, Devanarayana NM, Benninga MA, van Dijk M, Rajindrajith S. Psychological maladjustment and quality of life in adolescents with constipation. Arch Dis Child 2016; Epub ahead of print [PMID: 27402734]

264  Rajindrajith S, Devanarayana NM, Benninga MA. Constipationassociated and nonretentive fecal incontinence in children and adolescents: an epidemiological survey in Sri Lanka. J Pediatr Gastroenterol Nutr 2010; 51: 472–476 [PMID: 20562725 DOI: 10.1097/MPG.0b013e3181d33b7d]

265  Choung RS, Shah ND, Chitkara D, Branda ME, Van Tilburg MA, Whitehead WE, Katusic SK, Locke GR, Talley NJ. Direct medical costs of constipation from childhood to early adulthood: a population-based birth cohort study. J Pediatr Gastroenterol Nutr 2011; 52: 47–54 [PMID: 20890220 DOI: 10.1097/MPG.0b013 e3181e67058]

266  Kaugars AS, Silverman A, Kinservik M, Heinze S, Reinemann L, Sander M, Schneider B, Sood M. Families' perspectives on the effect of constipation and fecal incontinence on quality of life. J Pediatr Gastroenterol Nutr 2010; 51: 747–752 [PMID: 20706148 DOI: 10.1097/MPG.0b013e3181de0651]

267  Wang C, Shang L, Zhang Y, Tian J, Wang B, Yang X, Sun L, Du C, Jiang X, Xu Y. Impact of functional constipation on health related quality of life in preschool children and their families in Xi'an, China. PLoS One 2013; 8: e77273 [PMID: 24130872 DOI: 10.1371/journal.pone.0077273]

268  Swinburn BA, Sacks G, Hall KD, McPherson K, Finegood DT, Moodie ML, Gortmaker SL. The global obesity pandemic: shaped by global drivers and local environments. Lancet 2011; 378:804–814 [PMID: 21872749 DOI: 10.1016/S0140-6736(11)60813-1]

269  Teitelbaum JE, Sinha P, Micale M, Yeung S, Jaeger J. Obesity is related to multiple functional abdominal diseases. J Pediatr 2009; 154: 444–446 [PMID: 19874760 DOI: 10.1016/j.jpeds.2008.09.053]

270  vd Baan-Slootweg OH, Liem O, Bekkali N, van Aalderen WM, Rijcken TH, Di Lorenzo C, Benninga MA. Constipation and colonic transit times in children with morbid obesity. J Pediatr Gastroenterol Nutr 2011; 52: 442–445 [PMID: 21240026 DOI: 10.1097/MPG.0b013e3181ef8e3c]

271 Koppen IJ, Velasco-Benítez CA, Benninga MA, Di Lorenzo C, Saps M. Is There an Association between Functional Constipation and Excessive Bodyweight in Children? J Pediatr 2016; 171: 178–182.e1 [PMID: 26787379 DOI: 10.1016/j.jpeds.2015.12.033]

272 Driessen LM, Kiefte-de Jong JC, Wijtzes A, de Vries SI, Jaddoe VW, Hofman A, Raat H, Moll HA. Preschool physical activity and functional constipation: the Generation R study. J Pediatr Gastroenterol Nutr 2013; 57: 768–774 [PMID: 23857342]

273 Chien LY, Liou YM, Chang P. Low defaecation frequency in Taiwanese adolescents: association with dietary intake, physical activity and sedentary behaviour. J Paediatr Child Health 2011; 47: 381–386 [PMID: 21309885 DOI: 10.1111/j.1440-1754.2010.01990.x]

274 Roma E, Adamidis D, Nikolara R, Constantopoulos A, Messaritakis J. Diet and chronic constipation in children: the role of fiber. J Pediatr Gastroenterol Nutr 1999; 28: 169–174 [PMID: 9932850 DOI: 10.1097/00005176-199902000-00015]

275 Lee WT, Ip KS, Chan JS, Lui NW, Young BW. Increased prevalence of constipation in pre-school children is attributable to under-consumption of plant foods: A community-based study. J Paediatr Child Health 2008; 44: 170–175 [PMID: 17854410 DOI: 10.1111/j.1440-1754.2007.01212.x]

276 Carroccio A, Iacono G. Review article: Chronic constipation and food hypersensitivity--an intriguing relationship. Aliment Pharmacol Ther 2006; 24: 1295–1304 [PMID: 17059511]

277 Iacono G, Cavataio F, Montalto G, Florena A, Tumminello M, Soresi M, Notarbartolo A, Carroccio A. Intolerance of cow's milk and chronic constipation in children. N Engl J Med 1998; 339: 1100–1104 [PMID: 9770556]

278 Daher S, Tahan S, Solé D, Naspitz CK, Da Silva Patrício FR, Neto UF, De Morais MB. Cow's milk protein intolerance and chronic constipation in children. Pediatr Allergy Immunol 2001; 12: 339–342 [PMID: 11846872]

279 Gibas-Dorna M, Piątek J. Functional constipation in children – evaluation and management. Przegląd Gastroenterologiczny. 2014; 9 (4): 194–199. DOI: 10.5114/pg.2014.45099.

280 Tabbers MM, Dilorenzo C, Berger MY, et al. Evaluation and treatment of functional constipation in infants and children:

evidence-based recommendations from ESPGHAN and NASPGHAN. J Pediatr Gastroenterol Nutr. 2014;58(2):265–281

281   Fontana M, Bianchi C, Cataldo F, et al. Bowel frequency in healthy children. Acta Paediatr Scand. 1989;78(5):682–684.

282   Nurko S. Advances in the management of pediatric constipation. Curr Gastroenterol Rep. 2000;2(3):234–240.

283   van Dijk M, Bongers ME, de Vries GJ, Grootenhuis MA, Last BF, Benninga MA. Behavioral therapy for childhood constipation: a randomized, controlled trial. Pediatrics. 2008;121(5):e1334-e1341.

284   Tabbers MM, Boluyt N, Berger MY, Benninga MA. Nonpharmacologic treatments for childhood constipation: systematic review. Pediatrics. 2011;128(4):753–761

285   Epocrates. http://www.epocrates.com. Accessed April 3, 2014.

286   Biggs WS, Dery WH. Evaluation and treatment of constipation in infants and children. Am Fam Physician. 2006;73(3):469–477.

287   Nurko S, Youssef NN, Sabri M, et al. PEG3350 in the treatment of childhood constipation: a multicenter, double-blinded, placebo-controlled trial. J Pediatr. 2008;153(2):254–261.

288   Pijmers MA, Tabber MM, Benninga MA, Berger MY. Currently recommended treatments of childhood constipation are not evidence based: a systematic literature review on the effect of laxative treatment and dietary measures [published correction appears in Arch Dis Child. 2009;94(8):649]. Arch Dis Child. 2009;94(2):117–131.

289   Baker SS, Liptak GS, Colletti RB, Croffie JM, Di Lorenzo C, Ector W, et al. Clinical practice guideline: Evaluation and treatment of constipation in infants and children: recommendations of the North American Society of Pediatric Gastroenterology and Nutrition. J Pediatr Gastroenterol Nutr. 2006;43:e1–e13.

290   Loening-Baucke V. Polyethylene glycol without electrolytes for children with constipation and encopresis. J Pediatr Gastroenterol Nutr. 2002;34:372–7

291   Candy D, Belsey J. Macrogol (polyethylene glycol) laxatives in children with functional constipation and fecal impaction: a systematic review. Arch Dis Child. 2009;94:156–60

292 Candelli M, Nista EC, Zocco MA, Gasbarrini A. Idiopathic chronic constipation; pathophysiology, diagnosis and treatment. Hepatogastroenterol. 2001;48:1050–7

293 Mason D, Tobias N, Lutkenhoff M, et al. The APN's guide to pediatric constipation management. The Nurse Practitioner 2004; 29: 13–21

294 Holiday MA, Segar WE. The maintenance need for water in parenteral fluid therapy. Pediatrics 1957; 19: 23–32.

295 Coehlo DP. Encopresis: a medical and family approach. Pediatric Nursing 2011; 37: 107–12.

296 Bekkali NL, Bongers ME, Van den Berg MM, et al. The role of probiotics mixture in the treatment of childhood constipation: a pilot study. Nutr J 2007; 6: 17.

297 Banaszkiewicz A, Szajewska H. Ineffectiveness of Lactobacillus GG as an adjunct to lactulose for the treatment of constipation in children: a double blind placebo controlled randomized trial. J Pediatr 2005; 146: 363–8.

www.ingramcontent.com/pod-product-compliance
Lightning Source LLC
Chambersburg PA
CBHW061259220326
41599CB00028B/5713